# How to Reduce Overuse in Healthcare

A Practical Guide

Edited by

## Tijn Kool

## Andrea M. Patey

## Simone van Dulmen

## Jeremy M. Grimshaw

**WILEY** Blackwell

This edition first published 2024
© 2024 John Wiley & Sons Ltd

The right of Tijn Kool, Andrea M. Patey, Simone van Dulmen, and Jeremy M. Grimshaw, to be identified as the authors of the editorial material in this work has been asserted in accordance with law.

*Registered Offices*
John Wiley & Sons, Inc., 111 River Street, Hoboken, NJ 07030, USA
John Wiley & Sons Ltd, The Atrium, Southern Gate, Chichester, West Sussex, PO19 8SQ, UK

For details of our global editorial offices, customer services, and more information about Wiley products visit us at www.wiley.com.

Wiley also publishes its books in a variety of electronic formats and by print-on-demand. Some content that appears in standard print versions of this book may not be available in other formats.

*Library of Congress Cataloging-in-Publication Data*
Names: Kool, Tijn, editor. | Patey, Andrea (Andrea M.), editor. |
  Dulmen, Simone van, 1975– editor.| Grimshaw, Jeremy (Jeremy M.), editor.
Title: How to reduce overuse in healthcare : a practical guide / edited by
  Tijn Kool, Andrea M. Patey, Simone van Dulmen, Jeremy M. Grimshaw.
Description: First edition. | Chichester, West Sussex, UK ; Hoboken :
  Wiley-Blackwell, 2024. | Includes bibliographical references and index.
Identifiers: LCCN 2023008464 (print) | LCCN 2023008465 (ebook) | ISBN
  9781119862727 (paperback) | ISBN 9781119862734 (adobe pdf) | ISBN
  9781119862741 (epub)
Subjects: MESH: Low-Value Care | Medical Overuse | Patient Preference
Classification: LCC RA418 (print) | LCC RA418 (ebook) | NLM W 74.1 | DDC
  362.1–dc23/eng/20230614
LC record available at https://lccn.loc.gov/2023008464
LC ebook record available at https://lccn.loc.gov/2023008465

Cover Design: Wiley
Cover Image: © ArtHead/Shutterstock

Set in 10.5/13 STIX Two Text by Straive, Pondicherry, India
SKY10052474_080223

# Contents

# Preface

Low-value care refers to care that is not proven to provide benefits to patients or where benefits are small in relation to its harms and costs compared to alternatives (including doing nothing) and do not address patients' preferences. Over the last two decades, we have seen increasing global recognition of the existence of low-value care and its negative consequences. These include (direct and indirect) patient harms, unnecessary workload for hard-pressed healthcare professionals, wasted healthcare resources, and negative impacts on the climate. Low-value care may relate to both overdiagnosis and overtreatment. We are faced with major challenges such as demographic changes in societies globally with an increase in the elderly who often require healthcare, advances in biomedical discoveries that offer new therapeutic opportunities (but nearly always at increased costs), and human health resources challenges. There is an urgent need to address these challenges to protect patients, healthcare professionals and systems, and the planet.

In many countries around the world, healthcare professional societies have risen to this challenge by establishing Choosing Wisely and comparable programmes. These bottom-up professionally led campaigns have been highly successful in raising awareness about low-value care among healthcare professionals and patients and are increasingly feeding into professional training and quality initiatives. However, as we have observed in many other quality areas in healthcare, identifying a problem does not automatically lead to addressing this. The next urgent issue that we face is how to *de-implement* low-value care. This will be challenging because there are many drivers of low-value care at different levels of the system. Successful implementation will need careful diagnosis of the problem matched by targeted interventions that address important barriers and enablers. Successful de-implementation will require key actors, whether they are healthcare professionals, managers, policy makers, or patients, to change their decisions and behaviours, even whilst they are working, planning, or receiving care in time-poor, high-pressured, and somewhat chaotic settings. It can feel insurmountable to know how to start and what to do.

In this book, we hope to provide practical insights and tools to help those interested in de-implementing low-value care to systematically plan de-implementation programs. These build upon the insights and expertise of our multidisciplinary group of authors who have decades of experience in behavioural and social sciences and implementation and improvement research. We have tried to make this guide as practical as possible. We hope that this book will inspire and support healthcare professionals to take a first step in reducing medical overuse in their own environment and to continually learn from their efforts.

Tijn Kool
Andrea M. Patey
Simone van Dulmen
Jeremy M. Grimshaw

# Why Should We Reduce Medical Overuse?

Karen Born[1] and Wendy Levinson[2]

[1] Institute of Health Policy, Management & Evaluation, University of Toronto, Toronto, Ontario, Canada
[2] Department of Medicine, University of Toronto, Toronto, Ontario, Canada

## IT STARTED WITH QUALITY IMPROVEMENT

The idea that poor quality and patient safety harms are unacceptable and can be measured and improved was introduced into mainstream medical and public culture in the United States nearly 25 years ago and subsequently spread around the globe. This can be traced to the release of a ground-breaking report, *To Err is Human*, published by the Institute of Medicine (Donaldson et al. 2000). This report was part of a multi-year effort led by the Institute of Medicine to change the discourse around patient safety and quality in the United States. *To Err is Human* focused on the issue of medical errors and safety issues. It highlighted systemic drivers that lead to errors and established a patient safety

*How to Reduce Overuse in Healthcare: A Practical Guide*, First Edition.
Edited by Tijn Kool, Andrea M. Patey, Simone van Dulmen, and Jeremy M. Grimshaw.
© 2024 John Wiley & Sons Ltd. Published 2024 by John Wiley & Sons Ltd.

agenda with a focus on enhancing leadership, measurement, and systems to identify and decrease medical errors. It also highlighted that harm to patients from healthcare is a chronic threat to public health and is pervasive and preventable. This publication was followed shortly thereafter by the report, *Crossing the Quality Chasm*, which laid out an ambitious agenda for improving healthcare quality in the United States (Institute of Medicine 2002). This included establishing a six-dimensional framework to measure health system performance: safety, effectiveness, patient-centredness, timeliness, efficiency, and equity. In addition, *Crossing the Quality Chasm* offered three major categories for healthcare quality problems: overuse, underuse, and misuse. Overuse relates to healthcare services that have no benefits or for which harms outweigh benefits, underuse to healthcare services that offer benefits to patients but are not provided to relevant patients, and misuse to healthcare services that offer benefits in certain contexts but not others.

Subsequently, quality improvement collaboratives, campaigns, and efforts swept across the United States and other countries with wide variations in results and outcomes. About 14 years after the publication of *To Err is Human*, experts in quality and patient safety expressed frustration at the slow pace of change. In particular, decreasing overuse was rarely addressed by quality improvement efforts. The Institute of Medicine's report, *The Healthcare Imperative,* highlighted the shocking figure that nearly 30% of all healthcare costs in the United States were wasted or unnecessary (Yong et al. 2010). The report estimated that this unnecessary care, or overuse, costed upwards of $750 billion in 2009. The problem of overuse began to achieve more prominence as a quality problem, which necessitated further efforts to change. This figure of 30% of all healthcare being low-value has been reported in other high-income countries, including Canada (Canadian Institute for Health Information 2017). One commentary bemoaning the lack of change since the publication of the landmark reports over a decade earlier stated, in 2013, that, 'alongside important efforts to eliminate preventable complications of care, there must also be an effort to seriously address the widespread overuse of health services. That overuse, which places patients at risk of harm and wastes resources at the same time, has been almost entirely left out of recent quality improvement endeavours' (Chassin 2013).

This sentiment was supported by evidence that overuse is difficult to change. A United States study compared the quality indicators of overuse, misuse, and underuse in outpatient visits in 1999 and 2009 (Kale et al. 2013). The study found that during this period, 6 of the 9 underuse indicators improved, 1 of the 2 misuse indicators improved but only 2 of the 11 overuse indicators improved, with one getting significantly worse.

Chapters 2 and 3 will delve into why overuse is such a stubborn and challenging problem. And why strategies to reduce overuse need to be multi-pronged to be effective and supported by efforts to change the culture driving overuse, as well as systems that can drive overuse.

## THEN CAME A FOCUS ON OVERUSE

Overuse was originally defined in the Institute of Medicine reports, and since that time, there has been a proliferation of terminology to define and describe waste and overuse in healthcare. Common terminology includes low-value care, unnecessary care, appropriateness, overdiagnosis, de-adoption, and de-implementation. Table 1.1 offers four categories to classify key descriptions for overuse. Note that positive language, such as appropriate care, high-value care or right care, has been used to contrast with overuse and to emphasis quality problems associated with underuse and misuse, as well as overuse, and as such are not included in the table.

This book will use the terms overuse and low-value care as they are consistent with the broader language used in the quality and patient safety literature. However, clarity regarding terminology can help to communicate the complex topic of overuse to various audiences.

**TABLE 1.1** Overuse language and meanings.

| Category | Common terms | Application | Example |
|---|---|---|---|
| Processes of care which are not effective or cost effective | Unnecessary care<br>Low-value care<br>Waste<br>Inappropriate care | Processes of care that are not effective or cost-effective, delivery marginal clinical value or benefit to patients, and where harms outweigh benefits clinically | Annual or routine blood screening tests in asymptomatic patients |
| Overuse of a test, treatment of procedure | Overuse<br>Overprescribing<br>Overdiagnosis<br>Overtreatment | Variation in a practice across settings with additional use not delivering benefit | Overprescribing of antibiotics for respiratory tract infection in some settings or regions with similar case mix and population characteristics |
| Treatments which are no longer beneficial | Obsolete<br>Outdated technologies/care | A treatment which was once perceived to be beneficial but has been replaced with a better process of care, or now has strong evidence showing it does not work | Transfusing more than one red cell unit at a time when transfusion is required in stable, non-bleeding patients |

# OVERUSE AS A GLOBAL HEALTHCARE QUALITY CONCERN

In the chapter thus far, we have covered key American reports and data associated with the quality and patient safety movement. This movement spread globally, and with increased awareness of overuse came several key publications, which sought to describe and measure overuse in a global context. In 2017, *The Lancet* published a landmark special series of the journal with a focus on *Right Care* (Berwick 2017). The series emphasised the importance of the coexistence of overuse and underuse globally, offering evidence for overuse not just from high-income countries such as the United States, but also evidence of overuse in low- and middle-income countries. Also, the Organisation for Economic Cooperation and Development (OECD) released a report on overuse *Tackling Wasteful Spending on Health* in 2017. It began with a powerful statement contrasting spending pressures on healthcare systems globally with evidence that one-fifth of healthcare expenditures have no or minimal contribution to good health outcomes (OECD 2017). The OECD report linked the imperative to reduce overuse with the interconnected goals of spending less on healthcare while improving health. The OECD now includes overuse indicators, for example, antibiotic volumes, benzodiazepine prescriptions in older adults, and imaging tests in their annual *Health at a Glance* report (OECD 2021). The accumulation of evidence of overuse and presence of measures at the system level helped to articulate a case globally for the harms of overuse as a quality problem moving beyond costs. Importantly, these measures helped to emphasise a broad range of the harms of overuse to individuals to health systems.

It is important to frame and shape a narrative about overuse as going beyond wasteful healthcare spending to engage and motivate various stakeholders to take action. These include patients, clinicians, and the general public who may not be motivated to change due to government or payor concerns, but instead are concerned with individual safety and quality care (Born et al. 2017; Levinson et al. 2018).

Harms to individual patients from overuse include side effects from and medication interactions with unnecessary treatments, and incidental findings and testing cascades from unnecessary tests that can expose patients to risk. Overuse can also harm patients by wasting time or financial resources through delays in access to care, needless stress or worry, and wasted time and money pursuing follow-up appointments.

Harms to providers and organisations can be associated with wasted time, resources, and broader inefficiencies driving up wait times for patients and increasing inefficiencies for organisations. Inefficiencies in care, like pursing unnecessary test results, take up clinician time and can lead to excess workload and provider stress.

Overuse can harm healthcare systems at the regional, provincial, national, and indeed global level. Overuse wastes scarce healthcare resources. Public health crises, such as the opioid epidemic and antimicrobial resistance, are associated with and accelerated by the overuse and overprescribing of these medications. These can drive social and socioeconomic harms.

Finally, healthcare overuse is increasingly seen as harmful to human health and the environment (Barratt et al. 2022). There is a growing recognition of healthcare's climate footprint, the majority of which is driven by the complex supply chain of the manufacturing and distribution of healthcare goods such as pharmaceuticals, as well as service delivery in hospital and community settings (MacNeill et al. 2021). Recent reports suggest that healthcare sector emissions are responsible for nearly 5% of global net emissions (HCHW 2019). A key strategy to reduce healthcare emissions is to avoid overuse. The sustainability of any healthcare system depends on using resources to maximise benefit and avoiding wasteful spending that does not add value to patients or the public.

## WHAT CAN BE DONE TO ADDRESS OVERUSE?

With the accumulating evidence of overuse, as well as clear demonstration of the harms of overuse, increasingly efforts are being directed towards interventions to reduce overuse. Systematic reviews have highlighted that given the complexity of overuse, multi-component interventions that target both clinician and patient drivers of overuse are most likely to be effective (Colla et al. 2017). Components at the individual clinician and patient level, which draw from quality improvement approaches, include clinical decision support, performance measurement, and feedback, in addition to patient and provider education that is necessary but not sufficient to drive change. While health systems have explored policy initiatives to reduce overuse, including pay for performance, payment restriction, and risk sharing, there is limited evidence of effectiveness. Top-down approaches of payers to reduce overuse are often limited in scope and can meet resistance from both clinicians and patients if they are perceived as rationing healthcare.

## Choosing Wisely

National approaches to reduce overuse have been driven by various actors and groups, including payers and healthcare systems. However, the most well-known movement in the past decade has been a clinician-led approach to reduce overuse in nearly 30 countries globally (Born et al. 2019). *Choosing Wisely*® was initially launched as a campaign in the United States led by the American Board of Internal Medicine Foundation in 2012 (Cassel and Guest 2012). The campaign was aimed at galvanising physician leadership around ballooning domestic healthcare costs in the United States and lagging efforts to address overuse as an important quality problem. *Choosing Wisely* campaigns bring together national clinician specialty societies, which develop lists of recommendations identifying overused tests, treatments, and procedures within a clinical specialty.

*Choosing Wisely* campaigns share a core set of principles to ensure that clinician-led efforts to address overuse are not co-opted by government or other stakeholders. The campaigns should stay firmly associated with efforts to reduce harms to patients and improve quality at the individual, organisational, and health system levels. First, campaigns must be clinician-led (as opposed to payer- and/or government-led). This is important to building and sustaining the trust of clinicians and patients. It emphasises that campaigns are focused on the quality of care and harm reduction, rather than cost reduction. Second, campaigns must be patient-focused and involve efforts to engage patients in the development and implementation process. Communication between clinicians and patients is central to *Choosing Wisely*. Third, campaigns should be multi-professional, where possible, including physicians, nurses, pharmacists, and other healthcare professionals. Fourth, campaigns should be evidence-based wherein recommendations issued by campaigns are based on strong and high-quality evidence and reviewed on an ongoing basis to ensure credibility. Finally, campaigns must be transparent, so processes used to create the recommendations must be public and any conflicts of interest should be be declared (Levinson et al. 2015).

*Choosing Wisely* campaigns have been present for nearly a decade in some jurisdictions and the key question is whether these campaigns have an impact on reducing overuse. A measurement framework for *Choosing Wisely* campaigns was established which we will discuss in more detail in Chapter 7 on measuring low-value care. The framework suggests that campaign impact can be measured at three levels: first, awareness of overuse among relevant stakeholders; second, changes to processes in care; and third, changes to outcomes of care (Bhatia et al. 2015). These changes take time and involve changes to individual practice, as well as system drivers of overuse. A recent systematic review considering efforts to implement *Choosing Wisely* recommendations in the United States found that the publication and dissemination of recommendations through *Choosing Wisely* campaigns are necessary but not sufficient. Raising awareness and developing evidence-based recommendations will not address the complex drivers and factors associated with overuse; however, interventions by health systems and providers to implement campaign recommendations into practice using multiple components that target clinicians specifically, such as audit and feedback, changing order sets and education can reduce overuse (Cliff et al. 2021).

Efforts to reduce overuse need multi-component interventions due to the complex drivers of overuse. Overuse has been built into the culture of medicine for clinicians, and patients often believe that 'more is better' and underappreciate risks and harms of low-value tests, treatments and procedures (Kerr et al. 2017). Providers have developed long-standing practice patterns of the ways they typically investigate or treat particular conditions, often including exhaustive testing to rule out any potential but rare condition. Physicians learned to practice a particular way during their training, and changing these longstanding practice patterns is very challenging. Hospitals or clinics have systems that drive overuse, including order entry systems, routine order sets for hospital admissions or nursing directives for care, or routine annual visits and testing in primary care (Morgan et al. 2017). Healthcare systems create inefficiencies often due to the lack of integrated information systems, so redundant tests are done without providers knowing they had already been conducted. We will discuss all these mechanisms that operate on different levels in Chapter 2. Reducing overuse requires understanding the cause of the overuse in a particular situation and harnessing the appropriate mechanisms to drive change (Born et al. 2019). Changing the culture of overuse that pervades medicine is going to take years, and this journey is only in its early stages. This book gives readers a view of the present status of the problem, the opportunities and challenges of reducing overuse, and helps readers to start reducing overuse themselves.

## WHAT CAN YOU EXPECT IN THE FOLLOWING CHAPTERS?

This book consists of 14 chapters. In this first chapter, we have introduced 'overuse' and why it should be reduced. Chapter 2 describes why overuse exists. It is a multifactorial challenge with causes on several levels. Chapter 3 discusses the reasons why changing clinicians' and patients' behaviours, that is necessary for reducing overuse, is so hard.

In Chapter 4, we introduce a framework to reduce overuse that can help you to develop, evaluate, and scale up de-implementation interventions. In Chapter 5, we emphasise the importance of engaging patients in all the phases of the framework: designing an intervention and realising, spreading, and preserving the change.

In Chapter 6, we describe how healthcare professionals can start with reducing overuse by identifying potential areas of low-value healthcare and assessing the volume of low-value care to be de-implemented (see Chapter 7).

In Chapter 8, we describe how healthcare professionals can choose a specific strategy to reduce overuse by identifying the barriers for de-implementation and choosing the appropriate intervention for their identified problem (see Chapter 9). It is also important to evaluate the effects of an intervention to determine whether it was successful (see Chapter 10).

Then, we discuss the sustainability and spread of de-implementation interventions: how to increase the likelihood that interventions are sustainable and can be disseminated (see Chapter 11) and how to leverage professional education for sustainability and dissemination (see Chapter 12).

Finally, we present cases of de-implementation strategies from different countries through all abovementioned phases (see Chapter 13) and summarise how you can take steps to reduce overuse in your own practice (see Chapter 14).

## REFERENCES

Barratt, A.L., Bell, K.J., Charlesworth, K. et al. (2022). High value health care is low carbon health care. *Medical Journal of Australia* 216: 67–68.

Berwick, D.M. (2017). Avoiding overuse – the next quality frontier. *The Lancet* 390: 102–104.

Bhatia, R.S., Levinson, W., Shortt, S. et al. (2015). Measuring the effect of Choosing Wisely: an integrated framework to assess campaign impact on low-value care. *BMJ Quality and Safety* 24: 523–531.

Born, K.B., Coulter, A., Han, A. et al. (2017). *Engaging Patients and the Public in Choosing Wisely*. BMJ Publishing Group Ltd.

Born, K., Kool, T., and Levinson, W. (2019). Reducing overuse in health-care: advancing Choosing Wisely. *BMJ* 367.

Canadian Institute for Health Information (2017). *Unnecessary Care in Canada: Technical Report*. Ottawa, ON: Canadian Institute for Health Information.

Cassel, C.K. and Guest, J.A. (2012). Choosing Wisely: helping physicians and patients make smart decisions about their care. *JAMA* 307: 1801–1802.

Chassin, M.R. (2013). Improving the quality of health care: what's taking so long? *Health Affairs* 32: 1761–1765.

Cliff, B.Q., Avancena, A.L., Hirth, R.A. et al. (2021). The impact of Choosing Wisely interventions on low-value medical services: a systematic review. *The Milbank Quarterly* 99: 1024–1058.

Colla, C.H., Mainor, A.J., Hargreaves, C. et al. (2017). Interventions aimed at reducing use of low-value health services: a systematic review. *Medical Care Research and Review* 74: 507–550.

Donaldson, M.S., Corrigan, J.M., Kohn, L.T. et al. (2000). *To Err Is Human: Building a Safer Health System*. Washington DC: National Academies Press (US).

HCHW (2019). Health care's climate footprint. How the health sector contributes to the global climate crisis and opportunities for action. In: *Climate-Smart Health Care Series* (ed. H.C.W. Harm). Healthcare Without Harm.

Institute of Medicine, C.O.Q.H.C.I.A (2002). *Crossing the Quality Chasm*. Washington, DC: National Academy Press.

Kale, M.S., Bishop, T.F., Federman, A.D. et al. (2013). Trends in the overuse of ambulatory health care services in the United States. *JAMA Internal Medicine* 173: 142–148.

Kerr, E.A., Kullgren, J.T., and Saini, S.D. (2017). Choosing Wisely: how to fulfill the promise in the next 5 years. *Health Affairs* 36: 2012–2018.

Levinson, W., Kallewaard, M., Bhatia, R.S. et al. (2015). 'Choosing Wisely': a growing international campaign. *BMJ Quality and Safety* 24: 167–174.

Levinson, W., Born, K., and Wolfson, D. (2018). Choosing Wisely campaigns: a work in progress. *JAMA* 319: 1975–1976.

Macneill, A.J., Mcgain, F., and Sherman, J.D. (2021). Planetary health care: a framework for sustainable health systems. *The Lancet Planetary Health* 5: e66–e68.

Morgan, D.J., Leppin, A.L., Smith, C.D. et al. (2017). A practical framework for understanding and reducing medical overuse: conceptualizing overuse through the patient-clinician interaction. *Journal of Hospital Medicine* 12: 346–351.

OECD (2017). *Tackling Wasteful Spending on Health*. Paris: OECD Publishing.

OECD (2021). *Health at a Glance 2021: OECD Indicators*. Paris: OECD Publishing.

Yong, P.L., Olsen, L., and Saunders, R.S. (2010). *The Healthcare Imperative: Lowering Costs and Improving Outcomes: Workshop Series Summary*. National Academies Press (US).

# CHAPTER 2

# Why Does Overuse Exist?

Tijn Kool[1], Simone van Dulmen[1], Andrea M. Patey[2,4], and Jeremy M. Grimshaw[2,3,4]

[1] Department of IQ Healthcare, Radboud University Medical Center, Radboud Institute for Health Sciences, Nijmegen, The Netherlands
[2] Centre for Implementation Research, Ottawa Hospital Research Institute, Ottawa, Ontario, Canada
[3] Department of Medicine, University of Ottawa, Ottawa, Ontario, Canada
[4] School of Epidemiology and Public Health, University of Ottawa, Ottawa, Ontario, Canada

## A MULTIFACTORIAL CHALLENGE ON DIFFERENT LEVELS

To understand why overuse exists, it is important to understand the mechanisms behind overuse. Why do healthcare professionals order inappropriate laboratory tests and perform invasive procedures such as arthroscopies without evidence of necessity? And why do patients ask for harmful interventions and laboratory testing? Overuse is a multifactorial challenge with causes at several levels: healthcare professionals, patients, the clinical care context, healthcare organisations, and the healthcare system.

*How to Reduce Overuse in Healthcare: A Practical Guide*, First Edition.
Edited by Tijn Kool, Andrea M. Patey, Simone van Dulmen, and Jeremy M. Grimshaw.
© 2024 John Wiley & Sons Ltd. Published 2024 by John Wiley & Sons Ltd.

## Healthcare Professional Factors

Healthcare professionals play an important role in creating overuse. The lack of knowledge about current evidence of effective care may be a reason for providing low-value care. Healthcare professionals need to be aware of the scientific research of the effectiveness of treatments and its costs, but also of alternative treatment options. The general principle of good practice is that the healthcare professional uses scientific evidence as a basis for her professional practice. However, it is a challenge to keep an overview on all these alternatives. Adherence to guidelines and protocols by healthcare professionals is often modest (Grol and Grimshaw 2003).

The clinical behaviour of healthcare professionals involves two different processes: reflective and automatic approaches. Reflective processes are often described as reasoned behaviours based on knowledge about facts and values, whereas automatic approaches are described as routines or habitual behaviours and rely on heuristic decision-making (Strack and Deutsch 2004). Much of human behaviour uses automatic approaches to minimise cognitive effort and help people get through the day as these behaviours are typically the path of least resistance. Clinical actions are not different. They are often performed repeatedly, sometimes multiple times a day, in the same physical locations with the same colleagues and patients, under constant time pressure, and competing demands (Potthoff et al. 2018). We will elaborate on the behavioural aspects that may lead to overuse in detail in Chapter 3.

Healthcare professionals often make incorrect assumptions about patients' preferences and expectations resulting in patients being given unnecessary tests or treatments (for example, antibiotics for sore throats). If a patient does have a preference or expectation for low-value care, healthcare professionals need to discuss the lack of benefits and potential harms of the low-value care with the patient. This requires specific communication skills from healthcare professionals as illustrated in Box 2.1, which are rarely covered in professional education.

> **Box 2.1 Training of Communication Skills to Reduce Overuse**
>
> Doctors are aware that it is better not to prescribe antibiotics for a viral upper respiratory tract infection. However, they need the right conversation techniques to explain to patients why they send them home without a prescription. Training can help doctors to communicate better with patients and to talk with them about their expectations, values, and preferences. Training in shared decision-making led to less prescription of antibiotics for acute respiratory tract infections in primary care practice. Without this training, many doctors are afraid to disrupt the relationship with their patients if they refuse a certain intervention.
>
> *Source*: Adapted from Andrews et al. (2012) and (Coxeter et al. 2015).

## Patient Factors

Patients are increasingly encouraged to be empowered consumers who are well informed about different treatment options and actively participate in shared decision-making. The increasing availability of medical knowledge on the Internet (including social media) has increased the opportunities for patients to inform themselves. Therefore, patients' preferences, expectations, and values about care can influence what care they receive.

Patients may have unrealistic expectations about what healthcare services can actually achieve, partly because of unreliable information on (social) media. The media do not always provide information based on the latest scientific insights. Partly stimulated by uncertainty and the need to understand and relieve symptoms, patients might ask healthcare providers for a certain intervention, even if it is not effective. Many people assume, based on all kinds of media exposure and influences from their direct environment, that an extra check is always good and cannot do any harm. However, redundant screening can result in avoidable harm. Therefore, for example, clear age limits have been agreed upon in population-based screening programs. Providing reliable information to patients about the (lack of) added value of a test or treatment is very important, for example, patient versions of guidelines, as illustrated in Box 2.2.

## Box 2.2    Reliable Information to Reduce Overuse

Reliable patient information can have a major impact on healthcare consumption: in the Netherlands, a public information website on health issues (www.thuisarts.nl), developed by the Dutch College of general practitioners and based on their guidelines, is one of the best-visited websites in the country with approximately 220000 visits per day. Two years after the introduction of the website, primary care consultations had declined 12%, especially those by telephone, compared with no change in a control groups (Spoelman et al. 2016).

*Source*: Adapted from Spoelman et al. (2016).

## Preference for Acquiring Something

If the reduction of low-value care means that patients must stop with a treatment, for example, stop going to the physiotherapist regularly, this provides an additional psychological barrier. This is called the *endowment effect*: people value what they own more than what they do not possess (Thaler 1980). This mechanism could also work in the healthcare sector: patients highly value having something, in this case getting a test or treatment. This means that patients will not easily agree with no treatment as an alternative to the treatment they already receive, although doing nothing might be rationally the best solution.

## Clinical Care Context Factors

Factors in the clinical care context, such as the attitudes of the clinical team and the leadership of local healthcare providers, play an important role in the provision of low-value care. Culture and climate represent a social context composed of interpersonal networks that constrain and promote certain behaviours and interactions in the organisation where individuals work. Culture and climate are multidimensional and related concepts. Organisational culture includes the behavioural norms and expectations that guide the way workers do their work in a particular work environment. The organisational climate refers to the perception of the psychological impact that the work environment has on a worker's individual well-being and functioning (Aarons et al. 2012; Glisson et al. 2012). In Chapter 11, the role of culture in sustained effects will be described more in detail.

## Absence of an Open Culture

Team culture plays an important role in the provision of low-value care and maintaining the situation. For example, nursing teams explained performing inappropriate routine controls because their colleagues acted comparably (Verkerk et al. 2018). To change these habits and patterns, an open culture is needed that stimulates critical feedback. Also, for physicians, team culture plays a crucial role in deciding what activities they do and therefore also whether they provide low-value care practices. The dynamics of a group and the culture of a team are crucial in realising a climate in which overuse can be discussed. Therefore, a culture of trust is needed in which a safe, non-treating, blame-free environment ensures sense-making conversations between healthcare professionals. If such a culture of trust lacks, also in the patient–doctor relationship, healthcare professionals might be stimulated to provide low-value care and to avoid reducing overuse (Fritz and Holton 2019).

## Absence of Clear Leadership

It is also important that clinical leaders encourage and stimulate colleagues to adhere to guidelines and avoid specific low-value care. These clinical leaders can be direct colleagues in the team, but also, for example, representatives of professional or scientific associations.

## Healthcare Organisation Factors

Organisations in which healthcare professionals work may also contribute to overuse and low-value care. Local organisational procedures and protocols may not be aligned to the clinical guidelines or may obstruct healthcare professionals in restricting overuse. The working environment might be suboptimal for adherence to the so-called do-not-do recommendations.

The awareness of the culture in other organisations and stakeholders is also important for both de-implementing low value care and spreading de-implementation initiatives. Each organisation is unique, with its own culture, workforce mix, resources, and priorities. There is diversity in culture across different organisations, rendering a single formula for success unrealistic. Although some organisations may welcome the opportunity to de-implement low-value care to improve efficiency, optimise the use of limited resources, and reduce burden, other organisations may resist. Some organisations will be less likely to remove low-value care if it does not generate considerable revenue or if it prevents them from showcasing an innovation (albeit unproven or low-value) that gives them a competitive edge over other organisations. Organisations may also resist de-implementing low-value care that has a greater return-on-investment or revenue generating reimbursement structure, or among specialty health practices where health professionals may have fewer revenue streams (Verkerk et al. 2021). Fear of liability is another reason for organisations to resist supporting a culture of de-implementation. This may be particularly pronounced when it comes to reducing the frequency or intensity of delivering low-value care, for which it is less clear or even controversial to whom and when it would be considered low-value. Clear evidence supported by recommendations in clinical guidelines may tackle this barrier.

## Insufficient Time

An important factor that influences decisions in the consulting room is the way in which the work processes are organised. It is particularly important that healthcare providers have enough time to explain to patients why a specific test is low-value or stopping a treatment is appropriate (Buist 2015; Zikmund-Fisher et al. 2017). Doctors often report a lack of time as impeding the conversation with patients that is necessary for good shared decision-making. It is usually easier, and it takes less time to request a test than to convince the patient that this is not necessary (Kool et al. 2020).

## Lack of Coordination Amongst Healthcare Providers

Absence of good organisation and coordination between different healthcare providers, especially between primary care and hospital care, might stimulate overuse (Wammes et al. 2014). For example, multiple blood tests or other diagnostics are often performed, both in the primary care and hospital care, as a result of a lack of communication between the general practitioner and the medical specialist. It is important that information in the electronic patient records is available to different healthcare providers. In addition, because of a lack of coordination, patients might stay longer in the hospital than necessary, or their follow-up takes place in both the primary and hospital care.

## HEALTHCARE SYSTEM FACTORS

The way in which the healthcare system is organised may also facilitate the delivery of low-value care.

## Payment System that Rewards Volume

A payment structure such as the fee-for-service reimbursement creates a strong financial incentive to continue delivering low-value care. It emphasises volume as an important metric instead of value, and therefore, treatments of which the effect has not been proven are nevertheless reimbursed (Verkerk et al. 2021; Saini et al. 2017). Although this factor can be a key factor causing low-value care, it is important to realise that in many healthcare systems, some healthcare professionals have no or limited direct production incentives, such as nurses or primary care physicians, and still low-value care exists in these professions.

## Influence of the Pharmaceutical and Medical Device Industry

The pharmaceutical and medical device industry has a powerful influence promoting the use of their products that may stimulate unnecessary care (Verkerk et al. 2021). They influence decisions by healthcare professional through advertising, funding research, influencing guidelines, and organising education (Saini et al. 2017). The industry also influences political decisions by lobbying to increase product sales.

## Healthcare Insurance Policy

Financial incentives aimed at patients can work both in an impeding and stimulating way. When patients have a supplementary healthcare insurance, they might expect more from healthcare providers, for example, diagnostic tests, extensive treatments, or medication instead of waiting, or when this supplementary insurance will reimburse diagnostics or treatments without indication and with unproven effects. On the other hand, an insurance system with high co-payments for healthcare can lead to a reduction of healthcare consumption, because patients are more stimulated to consider whether a treatment is needed or not. This increases the room for doctors to discuss the added value of tests and procedures with patients.

**KEY POINTS**

- Overuse is a multifactorial challenge with causes on several levels.
- The levels are related to healthcare professionals, patients, clinical care context, healthcare organisations, and the healthcare system.
- Identifying influencing factors is important for the development of strategies.

# REFERENCES

Aarons, G.A., Glisson, C., Green, P.D. et al. (2012). The organizational social context of mental health services and clinician attitudes toward evidence-based practice: a United States national study. *Implementation Science* 7: 56.

Andrews, T., Thompson, M., Buckley, D.I. et al. (2012). Interventions to influence consulting and antibiotic use for acute respiratory tract infections in children: a systematic review and Meta-analysis. *PLoS One* 7: e30334.

Buist, D. (2015). Primary care clinicians' perspectives on reducing low-value care in an integrated delivery system. *The Permanente Journal* 20: 41–46.

Coxeter, P., Del Mar, C.B., Mcgregor, L. et al. (2015). Interventions to facilitate shared decision making to address antibiotic use for acute respiratory infections in primary care. *Cochrane Database of Systematic Reviews*, https://doi.org/10.1002/14651858.CD010907.pub2 CD010907.

Fritz, Z. and Holton, R. (2019). Too much medicine: not enough trust? *Journal of Medical Ethics* 45: 31–35.

Glisson, C., Hemmelgarn, A., Green, P. et al. (2012). Randomized trial of the availability, responsiveness, and continuity (ARC) organizational intervention with community-based mental health programs and clinicians serving youth. *Journal of the American Academy of Child and Adolescent Psychiatry* 51: 780–787.

Grol, R. and Grimshaw, J. (2003). From best evidence to best practice: effective implementation of change in patients' care. *Lancet* 362: 1225–1230.

Kool, R.B., Verkerk, E.W., Winnemuller, L.J. et al. (2020). Identifying and de-implementing low-value care in primary care: the GP's perspective-a cross-sectional survey. *BMJ Open* 10: e037019.

Potthoff, T., De Bruin, E.D., Rosser, S. et al. (2018). A systematic review on quantifiable physical risk factors for non-specific adolescent low back pain. *Journal of Pediatric Rehabilitation Medicine* 11: 79–94.

Saini, V., Garcia-Armesto, S., Klemperer, D. et al. (2017). Drivers of poor medical care. *Lancet* 390: 178–190.

Spoelman, W.A., Bonten, T.N., De Waal, M.W.M. et al. (2016). Effect of an evidence-based website on healthcare usage: an interrupted time-series study. *BMJ Open* 6: e013166.

Strack, F. and Deutsch, R. (2004). Reflective and impulsive determinants of social behavior. *Personality and Social Psychology Review* 8: 220–247.

Thaler, R. (1980). Toward a positive theory of consumer choice. *Journal of Economic Behavior and Organization* 1: 39–60.

Verkerk, E.W., Huisman-De Waal, G., Vermeulen, H. et al. (2018). Low-value care in nursing: a systematic assessment of clinical practice guidelines. *International Journal of Nursing Studies* 87: 34–39.

Verkerk, E.W., Van Dulmen, S.A., Born, K. et al. (2021). Key factors that promote low-value care: views of experts from the United States, Canada, and the Netherlands. *International Journal of Health Policy and Management* http://dx.doi.org/10.34172/ijhpm.2021.53.

Wammes, J.J., Jeurissen, P.P., Verhoef, L.M. et al. (2014). Is the role as gatekeeper still feasible? A survey among Dutch general practitioners. *Family Practice* 31: 538–544.

Zikmund-Fisher, B.J., Kullgren, J.T., Fagerlin, A. et al. (2017). Perceived barriers to implementing individual choosing wisely® recommendations in two National Surveys of primary care providers. *Journal of General Internal Medicine* 32: 210–217.

# CHAPTER 3

# Why Is It So Hard to Change Behaviour and How Can We Influence It?

Jill J. Francis[1,2,3], Sanne Peters[1,4], Andrea M. Patey[2], Nicola McCleary[2,5,6], Leti van Bodegom-Vos[7], and Harriet Hiscock[8,9,10]

[1] School of Health Sciences, The University of Melbourne, Melbourne, Victoria, Australia

[2] Centre for Implementation Research, Ottawa Hospital Research Institute, Ottawa, Ontario, Canada

[3] Department of Health Services Research and Implementation Science, Peter MacCallum Cancer Centre, Melbourne, Victoria, Australia

[4] Department of Public Health and Primary Care, the University of Leuven, Leuven, Vlaams Brabant, Belgium

[5] Eastern Ontario Regional Laboratory Association, Ottawa, Ontario, Canada

[6] School of Epidemiology and Public Health, University of Ottawa, Ottawa, Ontario, Canada

[7] Department of Biomedical Data Sciences, Medical Decision Making, Leiden University Medical Center, Leiden, The Netherlands

[8] Centre for Community Child Health, Murdoch Children's Research Institute, Melbourne, Victoria, Australia

[9] Health Services Research Unit, The Royal Children's Hospital, Melbourne, Victoria, Australia

[10] Department of Paediatrics, The University of Melbourne, Melbourne, Victoria, Australia

*How to Reduce Overuse in Healthcare: A Practical Guide*, First Edition.
Edited by Tijn Kool, Andrea M. Patey, Simone van Dulmen, and Jeremy M. Grimshaw.
© 2024 John Wiley & Sons Ltd. Published 2024 by John Wiley & Sons Ltd.

## THE CHALLENGE OF BEHAVIOUR CHANGE

To understand why healthcare professionals overuse tests and treatments, and why it is hard to change those behaviours, it is crucial to understand the principles that underlie behaviour change. What aspects of healthcare influence the opportunities for behaviour change?

### Is The Behaviour a Routine?

'The best predictor of future behaviour is past behaviour' is often regarded as a truism. In other words, repeated patterns of behaviour are resistant to change, and the more established those patterns are, the more resistant they are (Sutton 1994, Norman et al. 2000). This is not to say that the individuals who perform these behaviours are resistant; it is simply more difficult, more effortful, and more demanding to change an action if it has been performed before. In a clinical context, prescribing a particular antibiotic, ordering a specific blood test, and explaining a diagnosis to a patient are easier to do when they have been performed several times, as they are more likely to involve 'automatic processes', described in Chapter 2. Even if emerging evidence suggests that they are not required or should be done differently, the change itself takes extra thought, effort, and time, as 'reflective processes'.

### Is The Behaviour Rewarding?

Another well-known principle of behaviour is that we tend to perform behaviours that are rewarding, either intrinsically rewarding (e.g. makes me feel pleased or satisfied) or extrinsically rewarding (e.g. makes me rich). In the context of learning theory, these rewards are known as 'reinforcements', a reward that is conditional on performing the behaviour. What is perceived as reinforcement is very personal. For example, some physicians prescribe antibiotics to patients because they feel satisfied by fulfilling their patients' expectations (perceived or real), even though they are aware that antibiotics are of limited benefit in some circumstances (Md Rezal et al. 2015). Not prescribing antibiotics for those patients might lead to the risk of those patients seeking their healthcare elsewhere and may feel like a punishment (Md Rezal et al. 2015). Others, however, might feel pleased that they are reducing the risk of antimicrobial resistance and, therefore, decide not to prescribe an antibiotic if it is not required (Krockow et al. 2019). Clinical scenario 1 in Box 3.1 shows another example of the different ways of feeling rewarded in daily practice. Reinforcements can be experienced as something positive that is added to the situation in which a behaviour is performed, but it might also be that something negative is removed, for example, reducing anxiety. In the example of prescribing, some physicians prescribe antibiotics because they feel uncertain about a diagnosis (Md Rezal et al. 2015; Rose et al. 2021). In this case, decreasing the physicians' anxiety functions as a reward. In most circumstances, there are multiple interacting reinforcements at play. A healthcare professional who is already behind on their consultation schedule, for example, may decide to give the patient a prescription because it will be quicker than explaining why antibiotics are not necessary (Rose et al. 2021). Healthcare professionals might act differently when they encounter a patient who has a high level of health literacy and when there are not many other patients in the waiting room. When behaviour has a long history of reinforcement, it is particularly resistant to change. For example, a healthcare professional who routinely refers people for imaging to investigate lower back pain, and notices the relief that patients feel when their pain is taken seriously (the reinforcement), may find it difficult to recommend management options without imaging, such as physical therapy, weight reduction, or anti-inflammatory medications. A healthcare professional may not even be aware of the effects of these reinforcements. They can work at the 'automatic' level.

## Box 3.1   Arthroscopic Surgery in Degenerative Knee Disease: An Example of Behavioural Rewards

Clinical practice guidelines for degenerative knee disease advise taking medical history, conducting a physical examination and ordering radiography for diagnosis, and non-surgical treatment including pain medication, dietary advice, and exercise therapy. Surgery through a small incision in the skin using an arthroscope to detect, examine, and treat knee problems (knee arthroscopy) may be warranted only if the knee has a limited range of motion and if loose bodies, or meniscal tears, are present. Despite these recommendations, knee arthroscopy is still performed for many patients who will not benefit from it. It is difficult to stop performing knee arthroscopic surgery, as various reinforcements are applied. For example, orthopaedic surgeons want to help patients by reducing their pain and want to meet patients' expectations; some perceive pressure from patients for an arthroscopy and want to avoid losing those patients; and in many health systems, performing an arthroscopy is rewarded financially. In addition, despite the evidence, some orthopaedic surgeons believe that arthroscopy provides benefit, and they feel that it takes too much effort to explain to patients that the procedure is not needed. So, they proceed with the knee arthroscopy.

*Source*: Study from the Netherlands. Adapted from Rietbergen et al. 2020.

## Do Habits or Routines Play a Role in Sustaining the Behaviour?

Because reinforcements are delivered only if the target behaviour is performed, they occur *after* an action. Other important influences occur *before* an action is performed. These are 'cues' at specific times and in specific contexts, which trigger a specific behaviour. Examples are brushing teeth after breakfast or before bed, drinking wine after arriving home from a day's work, and buying a particular newspaper on the way to work. When a specific behaviour is triggered by a specific context, repeatedly, a 'habit' has been formed. Scholars have distinguished between *habits* and *routines*. *Habits* are triggered by contextual factors such as a patient with type 2 diabetes walking into the clinic, which triggers the physician's habit of checking the patient's blood pressure. *Routines* are sequences of behaviours, such as taking the patient's blood pressure while asking them how they have been feeling this week (Zisberg et al. 2007).

Developing habits and routines that are consistent with the clinical evidence makes it easier to give evidence-based care because they are relatively automatic and, thus, take minimal cognitive effort to perform. However, habits and routines that are inconsistent with the current evidence can be difficult to change, even when the healthcare professional is aware of the evidence, because they are embedded in established behavioural patterns and require effort to change. So, avoiding overuse (or *de*-implementation) of habitual behaviours can be even more difficult than initiating new clinical behaviours (implementation).

The problem with these habits and routines in the light of healthcare overuse is that these are driven by several cognitive biases, which, in general, stimulate healthcare professionals to perform more diagnostic testing and treatment. Examples of these biases are the preference for a sure and certain outcome over uncertainty, and the tendency to overestimate benefits and underestimate harms of diagnostic tests and treatments, which are often based on inaccurate perceptions of patient risk (Scott et al. 2017). Box 3.2 illustrates the many reasons for ordering too many laboratory tests and confirms that automatic processes can contribute to overuse.

## Box 3.2   Repeated Test Ordering: An Example of Habits and Routines from the International Literature

Laboratory testing is the highest volume healthcare procedures, and test results drive up to 70% of subsequent medical decisions (Forsman 1996). However, a synthesis of studies conducted in a range of countries showed that 15–25% of tests ordered are not clinically indicated (Zhi et al. 2013), representing wasted resources. Negative patient impacts can include pain, delays in appropriate tests, inaccurate diagnosis, and inappropriate treatments. Many hospital inpatients (40–45% in one study) receive tests daily regardless of whether the results indicate a potential problem, consistent with a culture of highly routinised testing influenced by past behaviour (Hure et al. 2019).

Additional factors also influence test ordering. Junior hospital doctors describe *erring on the side of caution* and over-ordering tests after being *caught out* (which feels like a punishment) when a senior doctor requests the result of a test that has not been ordered (Ericksson et al. 2018). Junior doctors also order tests when instructed by a senior colleague, even if this contradicts guidelines or their own views on clinical appropriateness (Ericksson et al. 2018). Primary care physicians have reported ordering tests to reassure patients rather than because of their own clinical suspicions (Houben et al. 2010). Finally, lack of relevant education, feelings of insecurity or uncertainty, and the ease of ordering via electronic systems also contribute to the persistent problem of inappropriate lab testing (Vrijsen et al. 2020).

*Source*: Review from Canadian Team.

## FOUR CRUCIAL QUESTIONS TO ADDRESS BEFORE WORKING TO SUPPORT BEHAVIOUR CHANGE

In relation to healthcare overuse, it would be unhelpful simply to 'admire' this problem without trying to find a solution. So, in this practical guide, we ask four questions:

- What is the specific (evidence-based) behaviour that needs to be adopted or embedded into practice? That is, if healthcare teams should do something differently, what is that different action, and who is responsible for doing it? For which patients? When and in what context should it be done? This can be specified using the Action, Actor,

Context, Target, and Time (AACTT) framework (Presseau et al. 2019). It is surprising that clinical practice guidelines may present a lot of information and evidence relating to a clinical problem but sometimes are unclear about these practical details (Michie and Johnston 2004). One simple way to reduce overuse in healthcare can be to specify precisely what should be done, using the AACTT framework. More information about the AACTT framework, and examples of its use, is presented in Chapter 8.

- What are the contextual factors that trigger the behaviour? Is the unnecessary care delivered in response to a patient request or the healthcare professional's assumption about what the patient wants? Or is there a shortage of equipment required to perform the evidence-based action? Is it too time-consuming? Careful attention to these existing factors ('antecedents') can identify how to change the behavioural triggers.
- What are the reinforcing factors that sustain the behaviour that needs to change as described above?
- Is there an evidence-based *substitute* action that could effectively replace the unnecessary action? (Patey et al. 2021; Helfrich et al. 2018; Patey et al. 2022b) Box 3.3 describes an example of offering a substitute action to healthcare professionals and patients.

## Box 3.3   The REMEDI (REducing MEDication in Infants) Study: Acid Suppression Medication in Infants: An Example of Behaviour Substitution

All babies cry with crying peaking around six to eight weeks of age. Some cry for more than three hours a day. Understandably, many parents are distressed by this crying and seek help from clinicians. For many years, such babies were diagnosed with gastro-oesophageal reflux and were offered treatments including acid suppression medications. However, acid suppression medications do not stop crying in otherwise healthy infants and, can even cause harm, such as an increased risk of gastro-enteritis, pneumonia, allergy, micronutrient deficiencies, and asthma (Gieruszczak-Bialek et al. 2015; De Bruyne and Ito 2018).

A research team worked with four hospitals in Australia to develop interventions designed to reduce unnecessary pre-scribing of acid suppression medication in babies. Baseline prescribing data were collected; interviews with parents and clinicians were conducted to understand why these medica-tions are prescribed and what could be done to stop prescrib-ing. These findings were then used to design and deliver a targeted behaviour change intervention to reduce medication use. Key to the intervention was providing clinicians with something else to do other than prescribing, i.e. behavioural substitution. Clinicians were trained and parents were pro-vided with leaflets on normal crying patterns and strategies to soothe and settle babies and reassure parents. These activities resulted in a 21% reduction in medication prescribing. Parents felt more confident to stop medication. Intervention resources are now freely available through state-wide clinical practice guidelines (Victoria 2021).

*Source*: Australian Study; Hiscock 2021.

## WHY IS IT SO DIFFICULT TO CHANGE THE BEHAVIOUR OF HEALTHCARE PROFESSIONALS?

There is substantial evidence that all the above principles influence everyone's behaviour, patients, members of the public, administrators, and healthcare professionals (Patey et al. 2022a). But arguably, healthcare professionals are different. And we need more than clinical knowledge to change behaviour. When people use an educational session to 'fix' healthcare overuse or try to persuade healthcare professionals that the evidence shows a particular practice should cease, they are making assumptions about knowledge deficits that are often unwarranted. In fact, in most investigations of healthcare overuse, there is already clinical consensus around what should be done, knowledge of individual healthcare professionals is already high, and they generally *intend* to do the evidence-based option. As well as the difficulty of changing habitual practice, there are several reasons why, despite sufficient knowledge and good intentions, healthcare overuse continues. Chapter 2 discusses many reasons at different levels. In the following section, we describe in detail the reasons on the level of the healthcare professional, in particular the automatic drivers that are resistant to behaviour change.

First, in any one encounter with a patient, healthcare professionals have many things to do, many potentially competing behaviours that need to be prioritised.

Second, healthcare professionals have been carefully trained to fulfil their professional responsibility with autonomy and to make complex decisions under pressure, even when there is uncertainty about patient needs.

Third, healthcare professionals are trained to take action (Doust and Del Mar 2004). So, doing nothing can feel wrong, and the reasoning around non-action can be difficult to explain to patients. In other words, *taking action* is part of the culture of healthcare.

Fourth, healthcare professionals tend to confirm their existing practice by noticing evidence that this practice is the best, the so-called confirmation bias (Lord et al. 1979; Driver 2001). This inhibits behaviour change because it reinforces the clinical behaviour if no negative outcomes have occurred and leads to being habitual as explained above.

Fifth, healthcare professionals tend to overestimate their adherence to evidence-based guidance. Research shows that there is a discrepancy of 27% between self-reported adherence and objective measurement of clinical behaviour (Adams et al. 1999). Moreover, healthcare professionals tend to overestimate the value of treatments, the so-called therapeutic illusion (Thomas 1978).

In general, there is a tendency of human beings to overestimate the effects of their actions, a tendency also referred to as the 'illusion of control' (Langer 1975). This overestimation is also legitimised by the importance that society attaches to healthcare and the opportunities of being treated for health complaints. These patient-related factors of continuing medical overuse have been described in Chapter 2.

Sixth, healthcare professionals, like many people, often fail to translate their good intentions into action. Research shows that intentions explain only 28% of the variance, on average, in future behaviour (Sheeran 2002).

Seventh, if healthcare professionals do not take action (even when that is consistent with the evidence), and something goes wrong, they are more likely to experience regret than if they did take action (Grimshaw et al. 2020). This asymmetry between 'action regret' (*At least I tried to do something for this patient*) and 'inaction regret' (*I did not do everything I possibly could have done for this patient*) is often a driver of healthcare overuse despite comprehensive levels of knowledge. Similarly, healthcare professionals' regret at not providing care that may benefit a few patients (regret of omission) overpowers their regret for providing unnecessary and potentially harmful care to many patients who never benefit (regret of commission). For example, consider a general practitioner who did not refer a younger woman for a screening mammogram who eventually died of advanced breast cancer. The general practitioner is likely to experience more regret for this omission than they do after referring hundreds of patients for a mammogram when it was either unnecessary or resulted in further invasive screening tests with subsequent negative results. In addition, such emotional and vivid cases come most easily to mind when considering a test or treatment. This cognitive bias is known as the 'availability heuristic' (Ubel and Asch 2015) and thereby also influences decision-making of healthcare professionals. This makes it more likely that healthcare professionals prefer action over inaction.

Eighth, they have a duty of care to patients that often coincides with a legal responsibility that needs to stand up to scrutiny, especially if something goes wrong. Related to this legal responsibility is the fear of accusations of malpractice, where consumers may sue their healthcare professional if they make a mistake. This can lead to defensive care. This means that requesting extra tests (confirmatory behaviour) or avoiding patients or procedures with a high risk (avoidance behaviour) may occur in order to reduce the chance of an accusation (Renkema 2017). Fear for these procedures can lead healthcare professionals to order tests or treatments that may be unnecessary but give them documented evidence in support of their clinical decisions (Verkerk et al. 2018).

Ninth, there are strong pressures for healthcare professionals to follow their colleagues' opinions and practices. Rather than explicitly consulting evidence-based guidelines, they often base their practice on internalised guidelines ('mindlines'), largely informed by their own and their colleagues' clinical experience updated through social interactions with opinion leaders and patients (Gabbay and le May 2004). However, clinical opinion has been described as the lowest level of evidence (Sackett et al. 1996). When a healthcare professional notes: *I recently treated a patient with intervention X; their condition improved and they were pleased with the care I provided*, they are drawing on experiential evidence that we know is flawed (Buchbinder and Harris 2021). Sometimes, for junior members of a clinical team, the powerful imperative to 'fit in' to the new team or to comply with established procedures can push the healthcare professional to adopt practices that they would not otherwise have done. For example, resident physicians conducting supervised visits in emergency departments use more resources when providing care than their senior colleagues, such as more frequent use of advanced imaging (Pitts et al. 2014). Conversely, juniors provide more readily evidence-based care than seniors, perhaps because juniors were more aware of the guidelines and less set in their ways (Hiscock et al. 2014). In addition, many healthcare environments are team-based, whereby providers from various specialties and disciplines work together to provide care. Such environments are often hierarchical, and therefore, the impact of social roles and power dynamics on clinical behaviour and quality of care need to be considered. For example, perceived hierarchies in the operating room are common barriers to effective communication in this setting, which contributes to the occurrence of adverse events for patients receiving surgery (Etherington et al. 2019).

Finally, healthcare professionals work in provider organisations that can limit the potential for practice change. For example, a healthcare professional's wish to avoid unnecessary preoperative test ordering may be thwarted by outdated policies and procedures that require all test results on a fixed list to be completed before an operating theatre can be booked for a specific procedure. Reducing overuse then first requires procedural change at the organisational level, which can involve lengthy consensus processes together with administrative or digital support to alter these established procedures. Organisational resources, structures, policies, and procedures are examples of contextual factors that influence whether or not an organisation is ready for change (Weiner 2009). Implementing complex organisational change involves collective action by many individuals and requires a degree of readiness for change. Organisational readiness for change refers to organisational members' *change commitment* and *change efficacy* to implement change in their organisation (Weiner et al. 2008; Weiner et al. 2009). Change commitment might be present because organisational members are willing to change (they find it valuable), because they have to change (they have limited autonomy), or because they feel they ought to change (Herscovitch and Meyer 2002). Change efficacy relates to organisational members' shared beliefs in their combined capabilities to prepare and deliver all actions required for achieving organisational change (Weiner 2009). Given that change involves a collective effort, problems might arise when some organisational members feel committed and capable, but others do not (Weiner 2009).

For all these reasons, there may be complexities around simply assuming that changing context or changing reward systems of healthcare professionals will change healthcare practice.

These additional challenges are evident in research demonstrating why, for example, reducing opioid prescribing for patients with chronic non-cancer pain is so difficult. Reducing prescribing for a specific patient involves multiple behaviours, including gradually reducing the prescribed dose, providing education about pain management and alternative treatments, and initiating referrals to support services. However, physicians struggle to conduct all these behaviours, reporting a lack of awareness of available services to refer patients to and a lack of time to deliver high-quality education (Kennedy et al. 2018; Desveaux et al. 2019). Initiating opioid reduction strategies for individual patients is a complex task. It requires physicians to balance the (often weak) guideline recommendations with their clinical experience, with many feeling that following guidelines alone risks destabilising patients, which can lead to the use of illicit drugs (Desveaux et al. 2019). Finally, initiating conversations with patients about tapering can introduce a perceived threat to the therapeutic relationship, which may prevent physicians from reducing opioid prescribing (Desveaux et al. 2019).

## DESIGNING INTERVENTIONS TO CHANGE BEHAVIOUR

Now, we have learned the opportunities and challenges of changing behaviour of healthcare professionals; we can start designing an intervention to change it. What is important while designing an intervention to change behaviour? How can we influence overuse in clinical contexts? And how do the answers to these questions relate to the advice provided in Chapter 2 about changing practice? These questions are explored in Chapters 8 and 9. First, Chapter 4 presents the Choosing Wisely De-Implementation Framework (CWDIF), a process framework that helps in selecting possible strategies and testing whether the strategy works. Subsequent chapters (Chapters 5–10) focus on each of the CWDIF steps, presenting tools, theories, and frameworks that are helpful for selecting and evaluating the evidence- and theory-based initiatives most likely to be effective in a particular clinical context.

## SUMMARY

- There are many reasons why it is hard to change the behaviour of healthcare professionals to reduce overuse.
- Changing established patterns of behaviour is difficult, even for healthcare professionals, and requires effort.
- This difficulty arises from competing clinical priorities, pressure to do something rather than nothing, expectations and rewards that are built into healthcare systems, and the relative ease of repeating actions that have been performed frequently in the past.

## SOURCES OF INFORMATION FOR SUPPORTING PRACTICE CHANGE AMONG HEALTHCARE PROFESSIONALS

- https://machaustralia.org/resource/implementation: a set of resources developed by healthcare providers in Melbourne, Australia, by the Melbourne Academic Centre for Health

## REFERENCES

Adams, A.S., Soumerai, S.B., Lomas, J. et al. (1999). Evidence of self-report bias in assessing adherence to guidelines. *International Journal for Quality in Health Care* 11: 187–192.

Buchbinder, R. and Harris, I. (2021). *Hippocrasy: How Doctors Are Betraying their Oath*. New South Publishing.

De Bruyne, P. and Ito, S. (2018). Toxicity of long-term use of proton pump inhibitors in children. *Archives of Disease in Childhood* 103: 78–82.

Desveaux, L., Saragosa, M., Kithulegoda, N. et al. (2019). Understanding the behavioural determinants of opioid prescribing among family physicians: a qualitative study. *BMC Family Practice* 20: 59.

Doust, J. and Del Mar, C. (2004). Why do doctors use treatments that do not work? *BMJ* 328: 474–475.

Driver, J. (2001). A selective review of selective attention research from the past century. *British Journal of Psychology* 92: 53–78.

Ericksson, W., Bothe, J., Cheung, H. et al. (2018). Factors leading to over-utilisation of hospital pathology testing: the junior doctor's perspective. *Australian Health Review* 42: 374–379.

Etherington, C., Wu, M., Cheng-Boivin, O. et al. (2019). Interprofessional communication in the operating room: a narrative review to advance research and practice. *Canadian Journal of Anaesthesia* 66: 1251–1260.

Forsman, R.W. (1996). Why is the laboratory an afterthought for managed care organizations? *Clinical Chemistry* 42: 813–816.

Gabbay, J. and le May, A. (2004). Evidence based guidelines or collectively constructed "mindlines?" ethnographic study of knowledge management in primary care. *BMJ* 329: 1013.

Gieruszczak-Bialek, D., Konarska, Z., Skorka, A. et al. (2015). No effect of proton pump inhibitors on crying and irritability in infants: systematic review of randomized controlled trials. *The Journal of Pediatrics* 166: 767–770, e763.

Grimshaw, J.M., Patey, A.M., Kirkham, K.R. et al. (2020). De-implementing wisely: developing the evidence base to reduce low-value care. *BMJ Quality and Safety* 29: 409–417.

Helfrich, C.D., Rose, A.J., Hartmann, C.W. et al. (2018). How the dual process model of human cognition can inform efforts to de-implement ineffective and harmful clinical practices: a preliminary model of unlearning and substitution. *Journal of Evaluation in Clinical Practice* 24: 198–205.

Herscovitch, L. and Meyer, J.P. (2002). Commitment to organizational change: extension of a three-component model. *The Journal of Applied Psychology* 87: 474–487.

Hiscock, H. (2021). Reducing medication in infants. www.rch.org.au/hsru/research/Reducing_medications_in_infants (accessed 15 June 2022).

Hiscock, H., Perera, P., McLean, K., et al. (2014). Variation in paediatric clinical practice: An Evidence Check review brokered by the Sax Institute (www.saxinstitute.org.au) for NSW Kids and Families. www.saxinstitute.org.au/wp-content/uploads/PAEDIATRIC-CLINICAL-VARIATION-ECHECK.pdf

Houben, P.H., Winkens, R.A., van der Weijden, T. et al. (2010). Reasons for ordering laboratory tests and relationship with frequency of abnormal results. *Scandinavian Journal of Primary Health Care* 28: 18–23.

Hure, A., Palazzi, K., Peel, R. et al. (2019). Identifying low value pathology test ordering in hospitalised patients: a retrospective cohort study across two hospitals. *Pathology* 51: 621–627.

Kennedy, L.C., Binswanger, I.A., Mueller, S.R. et al. (2018). "Those conversations in my experience Don't go well": a qualitative study of primary care provider experiences tapering long-term opioid medications. *Pain Medicine* 19: 2201–2211.

Krockow, E.M., Colman, A.M., Chattoe-Brown, E. et al. (2019). Balancing the risks to individual and society: a systematic review and synthesis of qualitative research on antibiotic prescribing behaviour in hospitals. *The Journal of Hospital Infection* 101: 428–439.

Langer, E. (1975). The illusion of control. *Journal of Personality and Social Psychology* 32: 311–328.

Lord, C., Ross, L., and Lepper, M. (1979). Biased assimilation and attitude polarization: the effects of prior theories on subsequently considered evidence. *Social and Personality Psychology Compass* 37: 2098–2109.

Md Rezal, R.S., Hassali, M.A., Alrasheedy, A.A. et al. (2015). Physicians' knowledge, perceptions and behaviour towards antibiotic prescribing: a systematic review of the literature. *Expert Review of Anti-Infective Therapy* 13: 665–680.

Michie, S. and Johnston, M. (2004). Changing clinical behaviour by making guidelines specific. *BMJ* 328: 343–345.

Norman, P., Conner, M.T., and Bell, R. (2000). The theory of planned behaviour and exercise: evidence for the moderating role of past behaviour. *British Journal of Health Psychology* 5: 249–261.

Patey, A.M., Grimshaw, J.M., and Francis, J.J. (2021). Changing behaviour, 'more or less': do implementation and de-implementation interventions include different behaviour change techniques? *Implementation Science* 16: 20.

Patey, A.M., Fontaine, G., Francis, J.J. et al. (2022a). Healthcare professional behaviour: health impact, prevalence of evidence-based behaviours, correlates and interventions. *Psychology & Health* 1–29.

Patey, A.M., Grimshaw, J.M., and Francis, J.J. (2022b). The big six: key principles for effective use of behavior substitution in interventions to de-implement low-value care. *JBI Evidence Implementation* https:// doi.org/10.1097/XEB.0000000000000351.

Pitts, S.R., Morgan, S.R., Schrager, J.D. et al. (2014). Emergency department resource use by supervised residents vs attending physicians alone. *JAMA* 312: 2394–2400.

Presseau, J., McCleary, N., Lorencatto, F. et al. (2019). Action, actor, context, target, time (AACTT): a framework for specifying behaviour. *Implementation Science* 14: 102.

Renkema, H. (2017). Professionals' attitude and behavior in an account-ability context: the physician's case.

Rietbergen, T., Diercks, R.L., Anker-van der Wel, I. et al. (2020). Preferences and beliefs of Dutch orthopaedic surgeons and patients reduce the implementation of "choosing wisely" recommendations in degenerative knee disease. *Knee Surgery, Sports Traumatology, Arthroscopy* 28: 3101–3117.

Rose, J., Crosbie, M., and Stewart, A. (2021). A qualitative literature review exploring the drivers influencing antibiotic over-prescribing by GPs in primary care and recommendations to reduce unnecessary prescribing. *Perspectives in Public Health* 141: 19–27.

Sackett, D.L., Rosenberg, W.M., Gray, J.A. et al. (1996). Evidence based medicine: what it is and what it isn't. *BMJ* 312: 71–72.

Scott, I.A., Soon, J., Elshaug, A.G. et al. (2017). Countering cognitive biases in minimising low value care. *The Medical Journal of Australia* 206: 407–411.

Sheeran, P. (2002). Intention – behavior relations: a conceptual and empirical review. *European Review of Social Psychology* 12: 1–36.

Sutton, S. (1994). The past predicts the future: interpreting behaviour–behaviour relationships in social psychological models of health behaviour. In: *Social Psychology and Health: European Perspectives* (ed. D.R. Rutter and L. Quine). Avebury: Ashgate Publishing Co.

Thomas, K. (1978). The consultation and the therapeutic illusion. *British Medical Journal* 1: 1327–1328.

Ubel, P.A. and Asch, D.A. (2015). Creating value in health by under-standing and overcoming resistance to de-innovation. *Health Affairs* 34: 239–244.

Verkerk, E.W., Huisman-de Waal, G., Vermeulen, H. et al. (2018). Low-value care in nursing: a systematic assessment of clinical practice guidelines. *International Journal of Nursing Studies* 87: 34–39.

Victoria, C.o.C.E.-W.a.C.S.C. (2021). Reducing harm from acid suppression therapy in infants. https://www.bettersafercare.vic.gov.au/clinical-guidance/paediatric/reducing-harm-from-acid-suppression-therapy-in-infants (accessed 15 February 2022).

Vrijsen, B.E.L., Naaktgeboren, C.A., Vos, L.M. et al. (2020). Inappropriate laboratory testing in internal medicine inpatients: prevalence, causes and interventions. *Annals of Medicine and Surgery* 51: 48–53.

Weiner, B.J. (2009). A theory of organizational readiness for change. *Implementation Science* 4: 67.

Weiner, B.J., Amick, H., and Lee, S.-Y.D. (2008). Conceptualization and measurement of organizational readiness for change: a review of the literature in health services research and other fields. *Medical Care Research and Review* 65: 379–436.

Weiner, B.J., Lewis, M.A., and Linnan, L.A. (2009). Using organization theory to understand the determinants of effective implementation of worksite health promotion programs. *Health Education Research* 24: 292–305.

Zhi, M., Ding, E.L., Theisen-Toupal, J. et al. (2013). The landscape of inappropriate laboratory testing: a 15-year meta-analysis. *PLoS One* 8: e78962.

Zisberg, A., Young, H.M., Schepp, K. et al. (2007). A concept analysis of routine: relevance to nursing. *Journal of Advanced Nursing* 57: 442–453.

# CHAPTER 4

# How Can We Reduce Overuse: The Choosing Wisely De-Implementation Framework

Jeremy M. Grimshaw[1,2,3] and Andrea M. Patey[1,3]

[1] Centre for Implementation Research, Ottawa Hospital Research Institute, Ottawa, Ontario, Canada
[2] Department of Medicine, University of Ottawa, Ottawa, Ontario, Canada
[3] School of Epidemiology and Public Health, University of Ottawa, Ottawa, Ontario, Canada

## INTRODUCTION

Since the start of the *Choosing Wisely* campaign, there have been some early successes in lowering low-value care through local interventions (Bhatia et al. 2015; Lin et al. 2016). However, there have been limited large-scale change (Rosenberg et al. 2015; Mafi and Parchman 2018). In the first years of the campaign, a lot of

*How to Reduce Overuse in Healthcare: A Practical Guide*, First Edition.
Edited by Tijn Kool, Andrea M. Patey, Simone van Dulmen, and Jeremy M. Grimshaw.
© 2024 John Wiley & Sons Ltd. Published 2024 by John Wiley & Sons Ltd.

attention was paid to making recommendations about which low-value care services should be reduced. However, we know that recommendations alone will not change clinical practice (Grimshaw et al. 2012; Nieuwlaat et al. 2013). How to de-implement low-value care and evaluate de-implementation initiatives has received much less attention. There is a lot of evidence and guidance on how to implement evidence-based strategies; however, few frameworks exist to guide the de-implementation process. Those that do exist focus on team culture or organizational change (Parchman et al. 2017) or target change in a specific clinical setting (Norton et al. 2018), making it difficult to generalise the frameworks across healthcare settings and contexts.

In this chapter, we introduce the Choosing Wisely De-Implementation Framework (CWDIF; see Figure 4.1). This can be used in different clinical settings helping you to plan, develop, and evaluate de-implementation strategies to reduce low-value care. It is important to realise that the framework is informed by behavioural and implementation sciences. De-implementation interventions can be delivered at any level within the healthcare system: from the individual patient and healthcare professional, healthcare groups or teams, and organisations providing healthcare, up to and including the larger healthcare system, as discussed in Chapter 2. Successful de-implementation interventions require key actors (e.g. patients, healthcare providers, managers, and policy makers) to change their behaviours and/or decisions whilst working in complex and often chaotic healthcare environments. Interventions that require people to change the care they deliver can be effective with the application of behavioural approaches (Davies et al. 2010; Hrisos et al. 2008; French et al. 2012) as we have explained in Chapter 3. Behavioural sciences have informed methods for identifying factors that explain and drive behaviour. In addition, they help you to select strategies or techniques to address the drivers of behaviour and provide guidance about reporting behaviour change interventions (Craig et al. 2008; Michie et al. 2005; Michie et al. 2013; French et al. 2012).

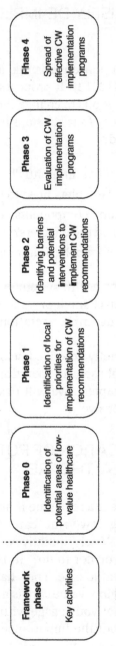

**FIGURE 4.1** The Choosing Wisely De-Implementation Framework. *Source:* Adapted from Grimshaw et.al. (2020).

## THE CHOOSING WISELY DE-IMPLEMENTATION FRAMEWORK

The framework builds upon an existing model by French and colleagues (French et al. 2012). It proposes a process to develop theory-informed interventions to change the behaviour of healthcare professionals involving four key steps in which four key questions should be answered:

1. Who needs to do what differently?
2. What barriers and enablers need to be addressed?
3. What intervention components could overcome the barrier and enhance the enablers?
4. How will we measure behaviour change?

The framework is not health system or country specific. You can use it for any initiative, small or large in scale, to systematically investigate better de-implementation strategies to reduce low-value care.

The framework is briefly described below with an example in the boxes of how each phase was operationalised in a Canadian example. In the next chapters, we will describe the phases (see Chapter 6–10) more extensively.

## PHASE 0: IDENTIFICATION OF POTENTIAL AREAS OF LOW-VALUE HEALTHCARE

Recognising that overuse is a real issue is an essential first step in the process of reducing low-value care. Several programmes, for example, Choosing Wisely initiatives, Smarter Medicine in Switzerland and 'To do or not to do?' in the Netherlands, have identified areas of low-value care. They have demonstrated that overuse in medicine and low-value care is a problem facing many countries. It is critical that you engage with decision-makers and healthcare providers about the importance of the overuse issue. They can actively contribute to the identification of low-value practices in their own discipline. This enhanced involvement of healthcare professionals can increase successfulness. We describe an example of this phase in Box 4.1 and in more detail in Chapter 6.

## Box 4.1 Application of the Framework: The Case of Unnecessary Preoperative Testing

### Phase 0: Identification of Potential Areas of Low-Value Healthcare

Many preoperative tests are routinely ordered for apparently healthy patients without any clinical indication (Munro et al. 1997). The subsequent test results are rarely used. In addition, unnecessary testing may lead physicians to pursue and treat borderline and false-positive laboratory abnormalities. The Canadian Anaesthesiologists' Society established its top five recommendations to reduce overuse, which focus on low-value tests in ambulatory surgery. They recommend that investigations should not be ordered on a routine basis, but should be based on the patient's health status, drug therapy, and with consideration to the proposed surgical intervention (Merchant et al. 2012).

## PHASE 1: IDENTIFICATION OF LOCAL PRIORITIES FOR THE IMPLEMENTATION OF RECOMMENDATIONS

Healthcare systems and organisations or clinics or individual clinicians should identify their own local priorities and focus on which low-value care practice(s) they want to de-implement. Not all recommendations are relevant for every region or institution, and it is not feasible to address all identified priorities simultaneously. Identifying priorities for implementation should be based upon data of the volume of the low-value practice in your setting. Also, professional consensus with stakeholder engagement is important and the recognition that there is a problem with low-value care in your setting. Finally, it is also crucial that there is robust evidence of lack of benefit of the low-value care you want to de-implement. The stronger the evidence of lack of benefit about a low-value practice behaviour, the better the opportunity to get consensus and avoid a debate that distracts from changing behaviour. An example of this phase is described in Box 4.2, and it will be described in detail in Chapter 7.

---

**Box 4.2    Application of the Framework: The Case of Unnecessary Preoperative Testing**

**Phase 1: Identification of Local Priorities for the Implementation of Choosing Wisely Recommendations**

Key health system leaders in Ontario (a Canadian province) met to identify initial overuse priorities to de-implement. A key initial hospital priority was preoperative testing prior to ambulatory surgery. Using administrative data from the Institute of Clinical Evaluative Sciences, a population-based study demonstrated the overuse of low-value tests and a significant inter-hospital variation across 137 Ontario hospitals. For example, 31% of patients received an electrocardiograph (ECG) with 26-fold variation in Ontario hospitals (Kirkham et al. 2015).

---

## PHASE 2: IDENTIFICATION OF BARRIERS AND ENABLERS TO IMPLEMENTING RECOMMENDATIONS AND POTENTIAL INTERVENTIONS TO OVERCOME THESE

Reducing low-value care will require a number of people to change their behaviours, the largest group being clinicians (French et al. 2012). Adopting a behavioural approach to de-implementing low-value care broadens the theories, methods, and tools available to promote this change. In Chapters 8 and 9, we will help you to choose the right theories and interventions to change a specific behaviour. Interventions using theories and methods from behaviour sciences can also target the environments in which healthcare professionals work, such as the system, the organisation and its policy, and their teams (Sniehotta et al. 2017). A key step when designing a de-implementation strategy is to assess the drivers of current low-value care and the barriers and enablers to de-implementing low-value care. The information about drivers, barriers, and enablers can then be used to inform the design of de-implementation intervention.

When designing interventions, you should consider:

1. What are the best intervention components or strategies to address the barriers?
2. What is the best way to deliver these intervention components or strategies?
3. How best to operationalise the components or strategies in the intervention?

By systematically answering these questions and identifying the most appropriate strategies to specifically address the barriers identified, you will increase the likelihood that the designed intervention will indeed change the targeted clinical behaviour(s).

There are a wide range of strategies available to reduce low-value care but no 'magic bullet' or ideal intervention can be used across all de-implementation initiatives. Evidence shows that all available strategies work some of the time, none work all the time, the observed effects are often modest, and it is not always clear why this is the case (Grimshaw et al. 2012). An example of this phase is described in Box 4.3, and it will be described in detail in Chapters 8 and 9.

## Box 4.3    Application of the Framework: The Case of Unnecessary Preoperative Testing

### Phase 2: Identification of Barriers to Implementing Recommendations and Potential Interventions to Overcome These

A study with Ontario anaesthesiologists and surgeons identified key beliefs associated with overuse of preoperative tests (Patey et al. 2012). Findings included conflicting comments about who was responsible for the test ordering, inability to cancel tests ordered by fellow physicians, and the problem with tests being completed before the anaesthesiologists see the patient. There were also concerns that not testing might be associated with harms (overnight admissions and readmissions) (Patey et al. 2012). These findings led to the development of a pilot intervention, which focused on increasing accountability in the healthcare system for preoperative test ordering.

## PHASE 3: EVALUATION OF THE IMPLEMENTATION

Given the relative lack of attention that has been paid to reducing low-value health, it is important that you evaluate new initiatives to generate knowledge about the effects of such interventions and how they work. In general, cluster randomised controlled trials are the gold standard for evaluating interventions (Eccles et al. 2003). But there are other study designs that may better suit your clinical setting like interrupted time series or a pre-post design. In Chapter 10, we will explain how you can evaluate your de-implementation intervention to reduce medical overuse.

Results from these evaluations will tell you whether an intervention was effective but not how and why the intervention was effective. In the absence of a theory-based approach, it may be difficult to interpret positive or negative effects of interventions or the failure of an intervention to bring about change (Eccles et al. 2005). You may also want to consider other types of investigations in addition to testing if the intervention works or not. This will increase the value of evaluating just the intervention alone. These studies can include *fidelity studies* to determine whether the content of interventions was delivered as intended. Also, *process evaluations* can be used to determine whether your intervention worked in the way you thought it would work. Interviewing participants will help you assess whether your intervention was sufficient to change participants' behaviours and understand participants' experiences of being part of the de-implementation initiative (Moore et al. 2022).

Given the limited resources for healthcare, you may want to assess the value for money of your de-implementation project to show your senior management the economic benefits of you intervention. Economic evaluation provides a useful framework to inform de-implementation decisions because it can synthesise data from various sources. It can also provide explicit estimates of long-term costs and benefits of alternative de-implementation interventions. Such an evaluation can address the uncertainty around costs and benefits as well as the decision-maker's dilemma. All these specific evaluations will be discussed in Chapter 10. Phase 3 of the Canadian example is mentioned in Box 4.4.

---

### Box 4.4   Application of the Framework: The Case of Unnecessary Preoperative Testing

#### Phase 3: Evaluation of The Implementation Program

A pilot study in one Canadian hospital of the proposed intervention developed from Phase 2 work (Patey et al. 2012) led to a 48% reduction in low-value preoperative ECGs. The intervention focussed on increasing accountability in the healthcare system for preoperative test ordering. Plans are underway to conduct a randomised trial of this intervention in 26 hospitals. In addition, fidelity studies, process evaluations, and an economic evaluation are planned alongside the trial.

---

## PHASE 4: SPREAD OF EFFECTIVE IMPLEMENTATION PROGRAMS

Providing detailed implementation information accompanied with stories of enthusiastic clinical leaders can help you ensure the spread of the positive results of the de-implementation intervention in other systems and regions (Levinson et al. 2018; Levinson et al. 2014). Engaging with knowledge users and other stake-holders throughout all phases of the framework will assist in the final phase. The goal of this phase is to help you encourage discussion on findings and future approaches for scale-up, spread of effective interventions, and generate thinking and action by those participating in this phase (Box 4.5). In Chapter 11, we will discuss how you can realise sustainable results of your intervention and which strategy to spread your results might be successful.

---

**Box 4.5   Application of the Framework: The Case of Unnecessary Preoperative Testing**

**Phase 4: Spread of Effective Implementation Programs**

Spread of the successful intervention to reduce the overuse of preoperative testing will include the development of a multi-jurisdictional learning platform for the sharing of methods and tools developed as well as training support for region to implement the intervention through the established Choosing Wisely Canada Implementation Research Network.

---

## KEY POINTS

- We present a 'how-to' framework for you to follow to de-implement low-value care in a systematic and rigorous manner.
- There are a wide range of strategies available to reduce low-value care, but no 'magic bullet' or ideal intervention can be used across all de-implementation initiatives.
- It is essential that efforts to de-implement low-value care utilise current state-of-the-science approaches and methods from implementation science and that healthcare systems maximally learn from initiatives to avoid unnecessary duplication of effort and waste.

# REFERENCES

Bhatia, R.S., Levinson, W., Shortt, S. et al. (2015). Measuring the effect of Choosing Wisely: an integrated framework to assess campaign impact on low-value care. *BMJ Quality and Safety* 24: 523–531.

Craig, P., Dieppe, P., Macintyre, S. et al. (2008). Developing and evaluating complex interventions: the new Medical Research Council guidance. *BMJ* 337: a1655.

Davies, P., Walker, A.E., and Grimshaw, J.M. (2010). A systematic review of the use of theory in the design of guideline dissemination and implementation strategies and interpretation of the results of rigorous evaluations. *Implementation Science* 5: 5908–5905.

Eccles, M., Grimshaw, J., Campbell, M. et al. (2003). Research designs for studies evaluating the effectiveness of change and improvement strategies. *Quality & Safety in Health Care* 12: 47–52.

Eccles, M., Grimshaw, J., Walker, A. et al. (2005). Changing the behavior of healthcare professionals: the use of theory in promoting the uptake of research findings. *Journal of Clinical Epidemiology* 58: 107–112.

French, S.D., Green, S., O'connor, D. et al. (2012). Developing theory-informed behaviour change interventions to implement evidence into practice: a systematic approach using the theoretical domains framework. *Implementation Science* 7: 38.

Grimshaw, J.M., Eccles, M.P., Lavis, J.N. et al. (2012). Knowledge translation of research findings. *Implementation Science* 7: 50.

Grimshaw, J.M., Patey, A.M., Kirkham, K.R. et al. (2020). De-implementing wisely: developing the evidence base to reduce low-value care. *BMJ Quality and Safety* http://dx.doi.org/10.1136/bmjqs-2019-010060.

Hrisos, S., Eccles, M., Johnston, M. et al. (2008). An intervention modelling experiment to change GPs' intentions to implement evidence-based practice: using theory-based interventions to promote GP management of upper respiratory tract infection without prescribing antibiotics # 2. *BMC Health Services Research* 8: 10.

Kirkham, K.R., Wijeysundera, D.N., Pendrith, C. et al. (2015). Preoperative testing before low-risk surgical procedures. *Canadian Medical Association Journal* 187: E349–E358.

Levinson, W., Kallewaard, M., Bhatia, R.S. et al. (2014, 2014). 'Choosing Wisely': a growing international campaign. *BMJ Quality and Safety* 003821.

Levinson, W., Born, K., and Wolfson, D. (2018). Choosing Wisely campaigns: a work in Progress. *JAMA* 319: 1975–1976.

Lin, Y., Cserti-Gazdewich, C., Lieberman, L. et al. (2016). Improving transfusion practice with guidelines and prospective auditing by medical laboratory technologists. *Transfusion* 56: 2903–2905.

Mafi, J.N. and Parchman, M. (2018). *Low-Value Care: An Intractable Global Problem with no Quick Fix*. BMJ Publishing Group Ltd.

Merchant, R., Chartrand, D., Dain, S. et al. (2012). Guidelines to the practice of anesthesia revised edition 2012. *Canadian Journal of Anaesthesia* 59: 63–102.

Michie, S., Johnston, M., Abraham, C. et al. (2005). Making psychological theory useful for implementing evidence based practice: a consensus approach. *Quality & Safety in Health Care* 14: 26.

Michie, S., Richardson, M., Johnston, M. et al. (2013). The behavior change technique taxonomy (v1) of 93 hierarchically clustered techniques: building an international consensus for the reporting of behavior change interventions. *Annals of Behavioral Medicine* 46: 81–95.

Moore, L., Guertin, J.R., Tardif, P.-A. et al. (2022). Economic evaluations of audit and feedback interventions: a systematic review. *BMJ Quality and Safety* 31: 754–767.

Munro, J., Booth, A. and Nicholl, J. 1997. Routine preoperative testing: a systematic review of the evidence. Health Technology Assessment (Winchester, England), 1, 1–62.

Nieuwlaat, R., Schwalm, J.-D., Khatib, R. et al. (2013). Why are we failing to implement effective therapies in cardiovascular disease? *European Heart Journal* 34: 1262–1269.

Norton, W.E., Chambers, D.A., and Kramer, B.S. (2018). Conceptualizing De-implementation in Cancer care delivery. *Journal of Clinical Oncology* 18: 00589.

Parchman, M.L., Henrikson, N.B., Blasi, P.R. et al. (2017). Taking action on overuse: creating the culture for change. *Healthcare (Amsterdam)* 199–203.

Patey, A.M., Islam, R., Francis, J.J. et al. (2012). Anesthesiologists' and surgeons' perceptions about routine pre-operative testing in low-risk patients: application of the theoretical domains framework (TDF) to identify factors that influence physicians' decisions to order preoperative tests. *Implementation Science* 7: 52.

Rosenberg, A., Agiro, A., Gottlieb, M. et al. (2015). Early trends among seven recommendations from the Choosing Wisely campaign. *JAMA Internal Medicine* 175: 1913–1920.

Sniehotta, F.F., Araújo-Soares, V., Drown, J. et al. (2017). Complex systems and individual-level approaches to population health: a false dichotomy? *The Lancet Public Health* 2: e396–e397.

# CHAPTER 5

# How Can You Engage Patients in De-Implementation Activities?

Stuart G. Nicholls[1], Brian Johnston[2], Barbara Sklar[3], and Holly Etchegary[4]

[1] Clinical Epidemiology Program, Ottawa Hospital Research Institute, Ottawa, Ontario, Canada
[2] Patient Partner, Choosing Wisely, Newfoundland and Labrador, Canada
[3] Patient Partner, Choosing Wisely, Canada
[4] Clinical Epidemiology, Faculty of Medicine, Memorial University St. John's, Newfoundland and Labrador, Canada

## WHAT IS PATIENT ENGAGEMENT AND WHY IS IT RELEVANT TO DE-IMPLEMENTATION?

The de-implementation of low-value care relies on both generating evidence about what does and does not work and then actively stopping low-value care in practice. These processes, and the results derived from the process, are contingent on several steps. First, how the question or topic is framed; second, how the issue at hand is understood, and the collection and review of evidence pertinent to informing the decision. Finally, it is shaped by how applicable that evidence is to practice. Involving patients, families, and caregivers in the prioritisation of topics, design of studies, and the implementation and spread of findings may improve success (Domecq et al. 2014; Shippee et al. 2015).

Unfortunately, patients, families, and caregivers may not be involved in any of these steps. In a recent analysis, only 6 of 136 clinician lists of the USA and Canada Choosing Wisely recommendations were found to have engaged patients or members of the public in their development (de Grood et al. 2022). This represents a failure to maximise the potential impact of recommendations, particularly given that evidence suggests that some campaigns have had limited impact on practice (de Grood 2020). Therefore, patient engagement is crucial in activities to reduce or de-implement low-value care. There are several studies of actual patient engagement in the de-implementation of low-value care as well as tools and resources to support your team at patient engagement.

Patient engagement is the meaningful and active collaboration with patients in governance, priority setting, conduct, or knowledge translation from an activity. Put another way, it is an activity done *with* or *by* patients, rather than *for*, *to*, or *about* them. Box 5.1 describes the most important terminology in patient engagement including the activities in which patient engagement can take place. However, you may also hear terms such as patient consultation, patient and public involvement, or public participation and the terms used locally may vary depending on where you are based (Abelson 2015; Banner et al. 2019).

---

### Box 5.1    Key Terminology in Patient Engagement

#### Patient

An overarching term that includes individuals with personal experience of a health issue and informal caregivers, including family and friends.

**Patient Engagement**

Meaningful and active collaboration in governance, priority setting, conducting research, and knowledge translation. Depending on the context, patient-oriented research may also engage people who bring the collective voice of specific, affected communities.

**Patient-Oriented Research**

Refers to a continuum of research that engages patients as partners, focusses on patient-identified priorities, and improves patient outcomes. This research, conducted by multidisciplinary teams in partnership with relevant stakeholders, aims to apply the knowledge generated to improve healthcare systems and practices.

*Source*: Adapted from CIHR Jargon Buster; CIHR 2022.

## MAKING A PATIENT ENGAGEMENT PLAN

Key to engaging patients within any de-implementation activity are questions regarding who will be engaged and when and how they will be engaged in the activity. We suggest that you develop a patient engagement plan (PEP) before starting any activity with patients (Etchegary et al. 2021).

An important first step when developing a PEP is to determine who you will engage. In some instances, you will be interested in a particular health condition, which may suggest patients with lived experience that may be valuable. Yet, other characteristics may also be important. While no one individual can reasonably represent a broader cohort of patients, it is important to be mindful of whether the patients engaged reflect the broad diversity of patients. For example, do your patients reflect the diversity of genders, ages, and ethnicities from your patient population? At the same time, you also need to identify individuals with whom collaboration is possible. This is not to say that individuals who challenge the status quo or pose difficult questions should be avoided, far from it. Rather, you need to have a respectful relationship – one that can raise questions, or critiques – but where discussion can occur. This applies to all parties; an unwillingness to listen and respect the perspectives of others will undoubtedly lead to conflict and failure.

To help identify patients and other stakeholders, we suggest you use a framework that provides a structure and avoids simply picking people you know. One example is the guidance developed by the Multi-Stakeholder Engagement Consortium. Their framework provides 10 factors, including expertise, influence, commitment, and time capacity, that should be considered when making decisions about which stakeholders are to be engaged (Parker et al. 2022). For example, does the engagement activity require specific lived experience of a disease or health condition? Key within this framework is the need to consider the training, support, and funding needs of those to be engaged. Do those engaged need an introduction to the area of interest, or perhaps the specific methodologies that will be employed? Will there be funding to support participation through honoraria? A failure to provide support or training options can lead to the exclusion of important perspectives.

A second element you should consider within the PEP is the stage(s) of an activity when you will engage patients. Here, we suggest using a simplified version of the Choosing Wisely De-Implementation Framework presented in Chapter 4 (Grimshaw et al. 2020). Figure 5.1 shows how you can engage patients in three areas: the prioritisation of topics, design of activities, and spread of findings from activities.

## The Level of Engagement

When developing a PEP, you will want to consider the level of engagement within each of the activity components. For example, what are the roles of patients who are being engaged? What are the expectations that will be placed on them? As above, we recommend using a guiding framework to structure discussion about

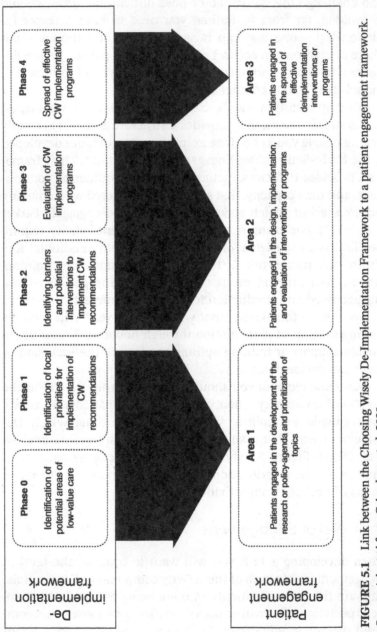

**FIGURE 5.1** Link between the Choosing Wisely De-Implementation Framework to a patient engagement framework.
*Source:* Adapted from Grimshaw et al. 2020.

the level of engagement. Figure 5.2 illustrates a research-adapted version of a common model. Within this framework, there are five levels of increasing engagement described as inform, consult, involve, collaborate, and support. While adapted for research, the levels can be applied to clinical activities, quality improvement, or research.

*Inform* is designated as the lowest level of engagement. Sharing information commonly reflects a base interaction in which there is one-way communication (usually) from an institution or a research team outward to the patient population or broader public. An institutional newsletter advising patients or the public of their research, clinical, or quality improvement activities would be an example of this level of engagement. Similarly, *Consult* may be viewed as a lower level of engagement in which a research team or healthcare organisation seeks input from patients or the public but retains control of that information and decides what to do with it. Focus group discussions or a survey of patient opinion would be an example of this level of engagement.

*Involve* and *Collaborate* represent more deliberative interactions in which patients are involved in the decision-making process and have some influence on final decisions and outcomes. In some cases, the level of engagement may be distinguished through terms such as *lived experience advisor* or *patient partner*. However, these terms are used inconsistently, and in practice, it may be difficult to distinguish the actual level of engagement from title alone. Consequently, it is important that you make clear the roles of patients and expectations of them so that they are clear about their level of engagement. Activities such as a patient advisory group or membership on a standing committee can be examples of involvement or collaboration.

Finally, *Support* relates to instances where the ultimate decision-making power is held by patients. Examples of support might include patients having decision-making control over which activities are funded or where they have final say within a research study. In practice, this may rarely be achieved within the context of de-implementation activities in healthcare.

| INCREASING STAKEHOLDER INFLUENCE ON THE RESEARCH → | | | | | |
|---|---|---|---|---|---|
| | **INFORM** | **CONSULT** | **INVOLVE** | **COLLABORATE** | **SUPPORT** |
| **STAKEHOLDER PARTICIPATION GOAL** | Researchers provide stakeholders with balanced and objective information to assist them in understanding the research. | Researchers obtain stakeholder feedback on the research. | Researchers work directly with stakeholders to ensure that stakeholder concerns and aspirations are consistently understood and considered in the research. | Researchers develop equal partnerships with stakeholders for undertaking the research. | Researchers provide input as requested to stakeholder-led research. |
| **PROMISE MADE TO STAKEHOLDERS BY RESEARCHERS** | We will keep you informed. | We will keep you informed, listen to and acknowledge your concerns and aspirations and provide feedback on how your input influenced the research. | We will work with you to ensure your concerns and aspirations are directly reflected in the research and we will provide feedback on how your input influenced the research. | We will include you as an equal partner in designing and conducting the research. | We will provide advice and assistance as requested to help you design and conduct your research. |

**FIGURE 5.2** Stakeholder engagement primer: 4. Options for engagement. *Source:* Adapted from Bammer 2021. Reproduced with the permission of Prof. Bammer.

Understanding the patient engagement needs of a de-implementation activity is important; not all projects will need to seek the same level of *support*. Indeed, you might have different degrees of patient engagement at different stages of your activity. Invariably, you will need more resources, time, and effort with higher levels of engagement. For this reason, it is important that you work through the levels of engagement in the planning stages of your activity (Etchegary et al. 2021). Costs can include compensation or honorarium to recognise the commitment made by your patients to support a de-implementation activity. You will also need to consider whether training is required for the research team or healthcare professionals involved. This might include training in patient engagement methods. You will also need to consider training or support for your patients. For example, would they need any background or training to facilitate their involvement? It is important that you develop an engagement plan at the outset and that the necessary resources are allocated at that time. Failing to do so will undermine the agreed engagement activities.

In the remainder of this chapter, we provide examples of patient engagement in de-implementation activities that we hope will provide context to the more abstract methodological discussion above. We then highlight important issues to consider when you engage patients. Finally, we provide resources that may prove useful. Throughout, we use 'patient engagement' as a general term that captures any activity on the spectrum from one-way communication to empowerment and support. Where we wish to note a specific level of engagement, we use the above terms as defined.

## Area 1 – Patient Engagement in Agenda Setting and Prioritisation

Engaging patients in agenda setting and prioritisation has two major benefits. First, you provide those most affected by the intervention with control over what will happen to them, supporting patient autonomy. Second, you facilitate the best use of limited resources by addressing the most important (health) needs of patients.

Agenda setting and prioritisation necessarily require you to adopt higher levels of engagement. At minimum, this usually requires *Consultation*, getting input from patients regarding what issues are most important to them about their health condition. It may likely require greater engagement to determine what a particular focus should be and the scope of the question to be addressed. To do this, you will need to adopt methods that allow or encourage two-way communication. Specific methodologies range from committee membership to more structured consultation using interviews, focus groups, or surveys. More deliberative methods that approach higher levels of engagement include multi-round Delphi surveys (Diamond et al. 2014; Nguyen et al. 2017) or James Lind Alliance Priority Setting Partnerships (Manafo et al. 2018).

Examples of patient engagement in agenda setting and prioritisation are perhaps those that are most readily available given the focus on developing lists of low-value activities within *Choosing Wisely* campaigns. Examples include the 'Thirteen things physicians and patients should question' developed by the Canadian Psychiatric Association (Canadian Academy of Child and Adolescent Psychiatry et al. 2017). The Canadian Psychiatric Association established a working group that *involved* representatives from professional societies as well as a person with lived experience from the Canadian Mental Health Association (see Box 5.2).

---

**Box 5.2    List of 13 Activities Identified as Low-Value Care in Psychiatry**

1. Do not use atypical antipsychotics as a first-line intervention for insomnia in children and youth.

2. Do not use Selective serotonin reuptake inhibitors (SSRIs) as the first-line intervention for mild to moderately depressed teens.

3. Do not use atypical antipsychotics as a first-line intervention for Attention Deficit Hyperactivity Disorder (ADHD) with disruptive behaviour disorders.

4. Do not use psychostimulants as a first-line intervention in preschool children with ADHD.

5. Do not routinely use antipsychotics to treat primary insomnia in any age group.

6. Do not routinely order qualitative toxicology (urine drug screen) testing on all psychiatric patients presenting to emergency rooms.

7. Do not routinely use antidepressants as first-line treatment for mild or subsyndromal depressive symptoms in adults.

8. Do not routinely order brain neuroimaging (computerised tomography or magnetic resonance imaging) in first episode psychoses in the absence of signs or symptoms suggestive of intracranial pathology.

9. Do not routinely continue benzodiazepines initiated during an acute care hospital admission without a careful review and plan of tapering and discontinuing, ideally prior to hospital discharge.

10. Do not routinely prescribe antidepressants as first-line treatment for depression comorbid with an active alcohol use disorder without first considering the possibility of a period of sobriety and subsequent reassessment for the persistence of depressive symptoms.

11. Do not routinely prescribe high-dose or combination antipsychotic treatment strategies in the treatment of schizophrenia.

12. Do not use antipsychotics as first choice to treat behavioural and psychological symptoms of dementia.

13. Do not use benzodiazepines or other sedative-hypnotics in older adults as first choice for insomnia.

*Source*: Canadian Academy of Child and Adolescent Psychiatry et al. 2017.

The American Academy of Paediatrics Section on Perinatal Paediatrics took a *consultative* approach in their work to develop a list of tests conducted on newborns and which may be subject to de-implementation. They asked family representatives attending an annual congress about the tests and treatments deemed low value. In the work of *Choosing Wisely Israel*, the Association of Family Physicians in Israel *consulted* patients regarding a list of tests and treatments family physicians should question. This was done by obtaining written feedback from patients on a newsletter article that detailed the recommendations as well as meeting with patients to have face-to-face conversations about the list.

Finally, patients were *involved* heavily in a prioritisation exercise conducted by the Canadian Rheumatology Association in determining its *Choosing Wisely* list of five items physicians and patients should question (Chow et al. 2015). Patients were involved not only in a working committee that generated a list of candidate items, but three patient members of the Canadian Arthritis Patient Alliance also reviewed evidence reports for each of the five candidate items.

## Area 2 – Patient Engagement in the Design and Conduct of De-Implementation Activities

Once priorities have been identified, you may also wish to involve patients in designing or conducting activities to reduce the use of low-value care. Approaches to engagement in this process can vary significantly. For example, some studies may conduct focus groups or other forms of consultation to get feedback on the proposed delivery of an activity. Other projects may maintain a patient advisor or advisory group who will provide input on an ongoing basis.

You can support this process by directly involving patients when developing your PEP. You can then work together to determine how patients would be engaged at different stages of the activity. For example, a team in Newfoundland and Labrador, Canada, reported how engagement varied across research stages, with written feedback sought on dissemination materials but more detailed discussion and *involvement* to develop the intervention and identify barriers to the delivery of the intervention. In *collaboration* with the researchers, the patients decided that they did not need to attend weekly operational meetings but would like to be *informed* of matters arising in order to maintain contact with the study team as the research developed (Etchegary et al. 2021).

You can also engage patients in key details of complex interventions. For example, in a study of adverse events due to polypharmacy in patients on haemodialysis, a research team developed a de-prescribing algorithm. Following the development of the original de-prescribing algorithm, three patient partners from Can-SOLVE CKD, a national network focused on research relating to chronic kidney disease, were *involved* in refining the algorithm. The patients informed the non-pharmacological options, directly informing how care may be managed (Lefebvre et al. 2020).

In another example, a research team *consulted* with a range of stakeholders, including patients, as part of study to reduce antibiotic prescribing in children. The team used focus groups to assess study feasibility and to shape the study design. This was enhanced with the *involvement* of a Parent Research Associate who was a core member of the team. This individual also led a Community Advisory Board made up of 15 parent, provider, and community stakeholders. The Parent Research Associate and Community Advisory Board had input into the study design, settings, participant burden, materials, procedures, interpretation of data, and dissemination of study findings (Goggin et al. 2018; Goggin et al. 2020).

## Area 3 – Patient Engagement in Spread

A key motivation for many patients to become engaged in research or quality improvement activities is to realise change in practice and ultimately improve care for others. By engaging patients in the sharing of your work, you will not only address the social obligation that research findings are made available (Bruhn et al. 2021), but you can also promote trust in the findings of your work. This has the potential to increase the uptake of those findings.

An integrated knowledge translation approach (Bowen and Graham 2013) is well suited to patient engagement given the explicit goal of engaging the range of relevant stakeholders – including patients – as partners in the activity. Your key stakeholder group will have the ability to bring about or influence change (Banner et al. 2019). This is particularly true when patients bring with them the ability to leverage organisations such as advocacy groups. Unfortunately, it seems that patients, families, and caregivers are less involved in these sorts of activities than with earlier stages such as setting the agenda or informing the intervention (Banner et al. 2019; Fergusson et al. 2018).

There are, however, some examples of patient engagement in the spread of de-implementation activities. One such example is the work by the Canadian Rheumatology Association Choosing Wisely Committee. In this case, patients from the Canadian Arthritis Patient Alliance and Consumer Reports worked with the research team to create plain language versions of the academic reports and helped to share the list with other arthritis patient groups as well as the broader public (Chow et al. 2015). Another example comes from *Choosing Wisely Italy* where members of two patient organisations (Altroconsum and Partecipasalut, meaning 'Participate in Health Care') have been involved as to make recommendations submitted by medical societies readable in order to help promote their dissemination (Kurdina et al. 2018).

## Important Considerations when Engaging Patients

We conclude this chapter with some important considerations that you should bear in mind when engaging patients in de-implementation activities. These considerations draw on both the published literature, as well as our collective experiences as researchers working to engage patients, as methodologists who support researchers, and our experiences as patient advisors who have worked with both clinical and research teams. For the interested reader, we suggest the 2018 review by Harrison and colleagues, which details foundational principles as well as a series of engagement best practices that cut across all stages of an activity (Harrison et al. 2019).

Our initial comment is that you need to be realistic in your expectations. Patient advisors or partners may have jobs, educational or caregiving commitments, or may simply not have the same workday as you. They may have to perform their tasks in evenings or at weekends. This may mean that they are unable to drop everything to contribute to your work on short notice or attend meetings during office hours. Similarly, patients may come with questions or may need time to build capacity and understanding around the engagement topic. Time should be built into your PEP to allow for this. Equally, while you may know that research or practice change can be a lengthy process, a key motivation for many patients is to see that change in practice. Exploring and addressing expectations of all engagement partners upfront is key.

Second, patient engagement requires resources, both human and financial. Plan ahead, and ensure that you budget time and resources accordingly. Things to bear in mind include the need for staff to liaise and communicate with your patients, reimbursement costs for travel and expenses incurred, as well as recognition for patient advisors or partners. While some individuals may wish to volunteer their time, recognition of the commitment is important as a show of respect and acknowledgement of the fact that engaging with research is not without cost. You can recognise patients in non-monetary ways, such as co-authorship on an article, or it can be monetary in the form of compensation or honorarium. Irrespective of the form of recognition, it is essential that you clarify the time commitment and form of recognition early in the engagement process.

Third, honest and open communication is important, even when there may be a lull in activity. There is nothing more demoralising than being asked for input that cannot be incorporated or that does not seem to go anywhere. In practice, we have found that this can be as simple as check-in emails to advise where things are with a project. A well-designed PEP allows you to decide what feedback and communication mechanisms will be used at each point during your project. For some activities within your project, you may send an email with key outcomes of a meeting. For others, you may have in person sessions to discuss project specific stages such as data collection or analysis. Whatever the method, ongoing and regular communication is critical for a successful patient engagement experience.

Fourth, it is never too late to engage patients, but the sooner the better; make time to talk to patients about your de-implementation activity – even if efforts are underway. There are likely activities or elements for which the patient perspective can still prove useful and insights that will be beneficial.

In addition to these practical steps, a key component to patient engagement is creating an environment that engenders trust and respect. It is important to recognise that patients will have a different perspective than clinicians, administrators, or researchers. It is precisely for this reason they will have been invited to the engagement activity. It is important for all other team members to acknowledge the patient's unique perspective and have an open mind with respect to contributions. You will likely hear personal stories about experiences. It is important to acknowledge and respect these, understanding that these can be traumatic experiences and where re-telling them can resurface that trauma. At the same time, a patient story is not their whole, and patients may bring other skills to the project such as lived experience of navigating a complex health system, or of managing fiscal issues.

## KEY POINTS

- Patient engagement is about meaningful collaboration: an activity done with or by patients, rather than for, to, or about them.
- Develop a PEP early and work with patients to establish how, when, and to what degree they will be engaged.
- Patient engagement requires time, effort, and resources but will improve the relevance and impact of your activity.
- It is never too late: a genuine approach to engaging patients will always be valued.

## SOURCES OF INFORMATION

### General Resources

Alberta SPOR SUPPORT Unit (2018). Patient engagement in health research: a how-to guide for researchers https://albertainnovates.ca/wp-content/uploads/2018/06/How-To-Guide-Researcher-Version-8.0-May-2018.pdf (accessed 16 February 2023).

Canadian Institutes of Health Research (CIHR) Ethics guidance for developing partnerships with patients https://cihr-irsc.gc.ca/e/documents/ethics_guidance_partnerships-en.pdf (accessed 16 February 2023).

The James Lind Alliance; Priority Setting Partnership https://www.jla.nihr.ac.uk (accessed 16 February 2023).

### Planning Tools

Vat, L.E. (2016). Patient and public engagement template. NL support: Newfoundland and Labrador's support for people and patient-oriented research and trials unit https://nlsupport.ca/getattachment/8dc1f539-d225-46fa-ba8d-2d06da934486/Patient-and-Public-Engagement-Planning-Template.pdf.aspx (accessed 16 February 2023).

SPOR Networks in Chronic Diseases and the PICHI Network (2018). Recommendations on patient engagement compensation https://diabetesaction.ca/wp-content/uploads/2018/07/TASK-FORCE-IN-PATIENT-ENGAGEMENT-COMPENSATION-REPORT_FINAL-1.pdf (accessed 16 February 2023).

George and Fay Yee Centre for Healthcare Innovation (2020). Patient engagement budget builder https://www.chimb.ca/s/2020-01-29_CHI_PE_Budget_Tool_v28.xlsx (accessed 16 February 2023).

## Patient Engagement Methods

George and Fay Yee Centre for Healthcare Innovation (2020). Methods of patient and public engagement https://static1.square-space.com/static/5e57d5337fe0d104c77cca10/t/5ed808e613338b 69dcb8f6df/1591216360358/20.05.20+PE+methods+of+Engage ment+web.pdf

Etchegary, H. et al. (2021). Operationalising a patient engagement plan for health research: Sharing a codesigned planning template from a national clinical trial. *Health Expectations*. http://dx.doi.org/10.1111/hex.13417.

## Evaluation Tools

Centre of Excellence on Partnership with Patients and the Public (CEPPP). Engagement Assessment Toolkit https://ceppp.ca/en/evaluation-toolkit

## REFERENCES

Abelson, J. (2015). Patient Engagement and Canada's SPOR Initiative. A Resource Guide for Research Teams and Networks.

Bammer, G. (2021). Integration and Implementation Insights. *Stakeholder engagement primer: 4. Options for engagement.* https://i2insights.org/2021/11/04/options-for-engagement (accessed 24 Apirl 2023).

Banner, D., Bains, M., Carroll, S. et al. (2019). Patient and public engagement in integrated knowledge translation research: are we there yet? *Research Involvement and Engagement* 5: 8.

Bowen, S. and Graham, I.D. (2013). Integrated knowledge translation. In: *Knowledge Translation in Health Care: Moving from Evidence to Practice*, 2e (ed. S.E. Straus, J. Tetroe, and I.D. Graham). Wiley.

Bruhn, H., Cowan, E.J., Campbell, M.K. et al. (2021). Providing trial results to participants in phase III pragmatic effectiveness RCTs: a scoping review. *Trials* 22: 361.

Canadian Academy of Child and Adolescent Psychiatry, Canadian Academy of Geriatric Psychiatry and Canadian Psychiatric Association (2017). Thirteen Things Physicians and Patients Should Question.

Chow, S.L., Carter Thorne, J., Bell, M.J. et al. (2015). Choosing Wisely: the Canadian rheumatology Association's list of 5 items physicians and patients should question. *The Journal of Rheumatology* 42: 682–689.

CIHR. (2022). *CIHR Jargon Buster* [Online]. Available: The Canadian Institutes of Health Research (Accessed september 2022).

Diamond, I.R., Grant, R.C., Feldman, B.M. et al. (2014). Defining consensus: a systematic review recommends methodologic criteria for reporting of Delphi studies. *Journal of Clinical Epidemiology* 67: 401–409.

Domecq, J.P., Prutsky, G., Elraiyah, T. et al. (2014). Patient engagement in research: a systematic review. *BMC Health Services Research* 14: 89.

Etchegary, H., Pike, A., Patey, A.M. et al. (2021). Operationalizing a patient engagement plan for health research: sharing a codesigned planning template from a national clinical trial. *Health Expectations* http://dx.doi.org/10.1111/hex.13417.

Fergusson, D., Monfaredi, Z., Pussegoda, K. et al. (2018). The prevalence of patient engagement in published trials: a systematic review. *Research Involvement and Engagement* 4: 17.

Goggin, K., Bradley-Ewing, A., Myers, A.L. et al. (2018). Protocol for a randomised trial of higher versus lower intensity patient-provider communication interventions to reduce antibiotic misuse in two paediatric ambulatory clinics in the USA. *BMJ Open* 8: e020981.

Goggin, K., Hurley, E.A., Bradley-Ewing, A. et al. (2020). Reductions in parent interest in receiving antibiotics following a 90-second video intervention in outpatient pediatric clinics. *The Journal of Pediatrics* 225: 138–145, e131.

Grimshaw, J.M., Patey, A.M., Kirkham, K.R. et al. (2020). De-implementing wisely: developing the evidence base to reduce low-value care. *BMJ Quality and Safety* 29: 409–417.

de Grood, C.M. (2020). *Patient, Family Member, and Public Involvement in Identifying Low-Value Clinical Practices for De-adoption: A Mixed Methods Study of Choosing Wisely Initatives*. MSc, University of Calgary.

de Grood, C., Sypes, E.E., Niven, D.J. et al. (2022). Patient and family involvement in Choosing Wisely initiatives: a mixed methods study. *BMC Health Services Research* 22: 457.

Harrison, J.D., Auerbach, A.D., Anderson, W. et al. (2019). Patient stakeholder engagement in research: a narrative review to describe foundational principles and best practice activities. *Health Expectations* 22: 307–316.

Kurdina, A., Born, K.B., and Levinson, W. (2018). Patient and public engagement in choosing wisely. In: *Toolkit*. New South Wales, Australia: Choosing Wisely Australia.

Lefebvre, M.J., Ng, P.C.K., Desjarlais, A. et al. (2020). Development and validation of nine deprescribing algorithms for patients on hemodialysis to decrease polypharmacy. *Canadian Journal of Kidney Health and Disease* 7: 2054358120968674.

Manafo, E., Petermann, L., Vandall-Walker, V. et al. (2018). Patient and public engagement in priority setting: a systematic rapid review of the literature. *PLoS One* 13: e0193579.

Nguyen, G.C., Boland, K., Afif, W. et al. (2017). Modified Delphi process for the development of Choosing Wisely for inflammatory bowel disease. *Inflammatory Bowel Diseases* 23: 858–865.

Parker, R., Tomlinson, E., Concannon, T.W. et al. (2022). Factors to consider during identification and invitation of individuals in a multistakeholder research partnership. *Journal of General Internal Medicine*.

Shippee, N.D., Domecq Garces, J.P., Prutsky Lopez, G.J. et al. (2015). Patient and service user engagement in research: a systematic review and synthesized framework. *Health Expectations* 18: 1151–1166.

# CHAPTER 6

# Identifying Potential Areas of Low-Value Healthcare-Phase 0

Moriah E. Ellen[1,2], Saritte M. Perlman[1], and Jeremy M. Grimshaw[3,4,5]

[1] Department of Health Policy and Management, Ben-Gurion University of The Negev, Beer Sheva, Israel
[2] Israel Implementation Science and Policy Engagement Centre, Ben-Gurion University of The Negev, Beer Sheva, Israel
[3] Centre for Implementation Research, Ottawa Hospital Research Institute, Ottawa, Ontario, Canada
[4] Department of Medicine, University of Ottawa, Ottawa, Ontario, Canada
[5] School of Epidemiology and Public Health, University of Ottawa, Ottawa, Ontario, Canada

## HOW TO IDENTIFY LOW-VALUE CARE?

The first step when addressing the challenge of reducing low-value care is to identify which aspects of care should be considered as low-value. The identification of low-value care focuses healthcare system and professional attention on them, facilitates measurement, and highlights opportunities for

*How to Reduce Overuse in Healthcare: A Practical Guide*, First Edition.
Edited by Tijn Kool, Andrea M. Patey, Simone van Dulmen, and Jeremy M. Grimshaw.
© 2024 John Wiley & Sons Ltd. Published 2024 by John Wiley & Sons Ltd.

de-implementation initiatives. Low-value care may be identified in many ways. Practice pattern studies identify and assess care among regions, organisations, or providers. These studies often show huge variation in tests, procedures, and treatments, in different disease states, at many risk levels, that might indicate low-value and, therefore, can be used as a tool to target interventions. For example, Kirkham et al. (2015) observed rates of preoperative electrocardiogram (ECG) and chest radiography for low-risk procedures in Ontario hospitals ranged from 3.4% to 88.8% and from 1.6% to 51.0%. Practice pattern studies may also observe the negative consequences of low-value care. For example, primary care patients receiving an ECG following an annual health examination are likely to receive further cardiology tests and consultations with no differences in cardiac events (Bhatia et al. 2017).

Randomised trials may demonstrate that a particular treatment is not effective or even harmful. For example, Vitamin D supplementation was found to be ineffective at improving cardiovascular risk (Veloudi et al. 2017). Comparative effectiveness research compares the benefits and harms of different interventions and strategies to prevent, diagnose, treat, and monitor health conditions in 'real-world' settings. The goal of comparative effectiveness research is to generate information that identifies the most effective interventions and that identifies optimal ways to implement effective care. De-implementation studies may demonstrate that low-value care can be stopped or reduced without adverse population outcomes. For example, three randomized controlled trials demonstrated no benefits of routine preoperative testing in patients undergoing cataract surgery (Balk et al. 2014). In general, when trying to identify low-value care, evidence syntheses of primary studies are more robust than single studies. It is important that recommendations identifying low-value care are regularly updated as new evidence emerges.

Identifying low-value care is often not clear-cut or easy. While some healthcare services have robust evidence about their effectiveness (or lack of it), the evidence base for many services is often more ambiguous. A service may be effective for some patients but not for others (Moore et al. 2019). For other aspects of care, individual patients may make different informed decisions about care options depending on their individual preferences about the associated benefits and harms. An example is weighing cancer treatment options based on the probability of being progression free for one year and the probability of experiencing varying levels of toxicity (Postmus et al. 2018).

Evidence 'grey zones' complicate the identification of low-value care requiring either identification of aspects of care that are always low-value such as ineffective or harmful treatments and/or specification of the patient groups and contexts when an aspect of care should be considered low value. For example, there may be high levels of bone scan use after routine prostatectomy for patients with prostate-specific antigen tests where the likelihood of a positive test was low (Kirk et al. 2019). There are still many examples of low-value care that are sufficiently clear-cut for healthcare systems to address whilst these challenges are worked through.

Even when there is clear-cut evidence about low-value care, there may still be stakeholder resistance to classifying aspects of care as low value and potentially discontinuing or limiting their use. This suggests that a key issue when identifying low-value care is the need to engage the necessary stakeholders during the process to improve the likelihood of a comprehensive, optimised, and successful process (Ellen et al. 2018). Information sessions such as town hall meetings, online modules, print publications, social media, and discussion forums are useful tools.

## Resources to Identify Low-Value Care

Identifying low-value care can be technically challenging and resource intensive, especially if you plan widespread engagement activities to ensure buy-in. Fortunately, there are several resources to help identify low-value care based upon evidence and experts' considerations. These include lists of recommendations identifying low-value and clinical practice guidelines and systematic reviews that may identify treatments and tests that are ineffective or harmful. Various groups globally are undertaking this work, which allows local initiatives to focus on de-implementation of low-value care. Below, we discuss these resources to identify low-value care, and at the end of this chapter, we give an overview in Table 6.1 with further information about these resources and further readings on each approach.

## Recommendation Lists

As discussed in Chapter 1, *Choosing Wisely* and similar initiatives initially focussed on developing lists of low-value care usually in collaboration with medical societies and professional organisations. Table 6.1 includes recommendations made by the Society of Hospital Medicine in 2022 as an example. Choosing Wisely Canada has recommendations in over 50 areas of healthcare (Choosing Wisely Canada 2022) (https://choosingwiselycanada. org/recommendations). Each area has between 3 and 13 recommendations that have been prioritised for immediate action.

The design of these bottom-up approaches aims to be healthcare professional-led, professionalism-based, and action-oriented. The process for developing recommendations generally includes soliciting input from professionals in the field about potentially unnecessary services, reviewing supporting evidence, and narrowing down and revising recommendations as necessary.

Once the list is refined, it is disseminated to members of the medical societies and professional organisations, and patients and healthcare systems more broadly. Ideally, alongside these initiatives to identify low-value care, medical societies and professional organisations can educate and engage their members to build awareness, involvement, and support for addressing low-value care. There are many resources available to engage in these processes and stay current with the body of knowledge, such as case studies, modules, success stories, analyses, guides, and toolkits. Much progress has been made by utilising these bottom-up approaches to help healthcare professionals and patients engage in conversations about low-value care and make smart and effective choices to ensure high-quality care.

## Clinical Practice Guidelines

Clinical practice guidelines are 'statements that include recommendations intended to optimise patient care. They are informed by systematic reviews of evidence and an assessment of the benefits and harms of alternative care options' (Institute of Medicine et al. 2011). The development of clinical practice guidelines provides further opportunities to identify low-value care and make recommendations addressing these. For example, the US Preventive Services Task Force explicitly uses a D grade when it recommends against a service and there is 'moderate or high certainty that the service has no net benefit or that harms outweigh the benefits' (USPSTF 2012). This allows for rapid identification of areas of low-value care. Identifying low-value care is often less explicit in guidelines produced by other agencies; nevertheless, guidelines can help identify low-value care especially if you are interested in a specific clinical area. For example, in the Netherlands, do-not-do lists for medical specialists, nurses, and general practitioners are composed based on recommendations in clinical guidelines (Wammes et al. 2016; Verkerk et al. 2018; van Dulmen et al. 2022).

## Health Technology Assessments

Health technology assessments (HTAs) are top-down mostly government-led assessments focusing on clinical and cost-effectiveness issues and their respective ethical, legal, social, and organisational challenges. The goal is to evaluate new health technologies and provide ongoing evaluation over the technology life cycle by conducting systematic evaluations by interdisciplinary groups. In addition to direct and intended consequences, HTAs highlight indirect and unintended consequences as well, such as demonstrating potential areas of overuse within the field of health technology. HTAs inform technology-related healthcare policy and can be applied to the identification of overuse within those policies and the utilisation of specific health technologies.

## Evidence Syntheses and Systematic Reviews

Low-value care can also be identified from evidence syntheses that bring together all relevant information on a research question, for example, the benefits and harms of a treatment, the performance of a diagnostic test, or patients' experiences of healthcare. There are thousands of evidence syntheses published each year, though unfortunately the quality and trustworthiness of evidence syntheses is variable (Mustafa et al. 2013). However, repeated studies have shown that evidence syntheses undertaken by Cochrane and published in the *Cochrane Database of Systematic Reviews* are of generally high quality. Cochrane is a global independent network of researchers, professionals, patients, carers, and people interested in health who work together to produce credible, accessible health information that is free of conflicts of interest. Those evidence syntheses can be used to identify low-value care although you need to look up reviews of specific topics of interest.

## From Identification to Measurement

Identification and measurement of low-value are interconnected. Lists identifying low-value care help prioritise what aspects of care could be measured to support local priorities for de-implementation. In the next chapter, we will describe how you can measure low-value care.

**TABLE 6.1** Processes and approaches to identify low-value care

| Process | Example | Further Reading |
|---|---|---|
| Choosing Wisely International | Society of Hospital Medicine – Adult Hospital Medicine (SHM 2022)<br><br>1. Avoid using opioids for treatment of mild, acute pain. For moderate to severe acute pain, if opioids are used, it should be in conjunction with non-opioid methods with the lowest effective dose for the shortest required duration.<br><br>2. Do not maintain a peripheral capillary oxygen saturation ($SpO_2$) of higher than 96% when using supplemental oxygen, unless for carbon monoxide poisoning, cluster headaches, sickle cell crisis, or pneumothorax.<br><br>3. Do not wake patients at night for routine care; redesign workflow to promote sleep at night.<br><br>4. Do not order creatine kinase or creatine kinase-myocardial band in suspected acute coronary syndrome or acute myocardial infarction.<br><br>5. Do not order daily chest radiographs in hospitalised patients unless there are specific clinical indications.<br><br>6. Do not routinely prescribe venous thromboembolism (VTE) prophylaxis to all hospitalised patients; use an evidence-based risk stratification system to determine whether a patient needs VTE prophylaxis. If they do warrant prophylaxis, use a bleeding risk assessment to determine if mechanical rather than pharmacologic prophylaxis is more appropriate. | https://www.choosingwisely.org/clinician-lists<br><br>Cassel, C.K. and Guest, J.A., 2012. Choosing wisely: helping physicians and patients make smart decisions about their care. Journal of the American Medical Association, 307(17), pp. 1801–1802<br><br>Levinson, W., Born, K. and Wolfson, D., 2018. Choosing wisely campaigns: a work in progress. Journal of the American Medical Association, 319(19), pp. 1975–1976.<br><br>Cliff, B.Q., Avancena, A.L., Hirth, R.A. and LEE, S.Y.D., 2021. The Impact of Choosing Wisely Interventions on Low-Value Medical Services: A Systematic Review. The Milbank Quarterly, 99(4), pp. 1024–1058. |

(Continued)

**TABLE 6.1** (Continued)

| Process | Example | Further Reading |
|---|---|---|
| Cochrane Collaboration | Airway clearance techniques for bronchiectasis (Lee et al. 2015) Chest physical therapy techniques did not appear to reduce the overall severity of disease for bronchiectasis but there may be reduction in the rate of progression of disease and improvement in the health-related qualities of life. Related Choosing Wisely recommendation: Do not routinely use airway clearance therapy in conditions such as asthma, bronchiolitis, and pneumonia. | https://www.cochranelibrary.com/cdsr/about-cdsr |
| US Preventive Services Task Force (USPSTF) | The USPSTF recommends against screening for pancreatic cancer in asymptomatic adults (2020) <br>• Impact on morbidity and mortality of screening for pancreatic adenocarcinoma is not well documented. <br>• There is insufficient evidence to assess benefits or harms of surgical intervention for screen-detected pancreatic adenocarcinoma (Henrikson et al. 2019) <br><br>The USPSTF recommends against screening for asymptomatic carotid artery stenosis in the general adult population (2022) <br>• No population-based screening trials of screening versus no screening for carotid artery stenosis have ever been conducted. <br>• Little indirect evidence exists regarding whether carotid revascularisation is superior to best medical management (Guirguis-Blake et al. 2021) | https://www.uspreventiveservicestaskforce.org/uspstf/recommendation-topics |

## Research efforts

**Comparative effectiveness research**

Addressing 'waste' in diagnostic imaging: some implications of comparative effectiveness research (Elshaug et al. 2010)

Five case studies:

1. Ottawa ankle rules

    Pretest risk assessment performed by an appropriately skilled clinician could avoid imaging in many low-risk patients who currently receive imaging.

2. Follow-up mammography

    Need better evidence for the value of surveillance mammography and for its indications

3. Imaging for low back pain

    Routine immediate lumbar imaging is not required in patients who present with low back pain without any clinical features to suggest underlying 'red flag' conditions

4. Routine chest X-rays in intensive care units

    An on-demand strategy can safely reduce the average number of chest X-rays per patient day of mechanical ventilation by 32% without increasing days on ventilation, length of stay in intensive care, or mortality. Furthermore, there was no statistically significant difference in the number of chest X-rays that led to diagnostic or therapeutic interventions

5. Screening mammography

    Overdiagnosis estimated to be higher for women at the younger end of the target screening population than for those at the older end

Sheridan, S.L., Sutkowi-Hemstreet, A., Barclay, C., Brewer, N.T., Dolor, R.J., Gizlice, Z., Lewis, C.L., Reuland, D.S., Golin, CE., Kistler, CE. and Vu, M., 2016. A comparative effectiveness trial of alternate formats for presenting benefits and harms information for low-value screening services: a randomised clinical trial. JAMA internal medicine, 176(1), pp. 31–41.

Padula, W.V., Berzon, R.A., Mujuru, P. and Meltzer, D.O., 2021. Comparative Effectiveness Research in Health Disparity Populations. The Science of Health Disparities Research, pp. 359–374.

(Continued)

**TABLE 6.1** (Continued)

| Process | Example | Further Reading |
|---------|---------|-----------------|
| HTA | Case study: surgical treatment of carpal tunnel syndrome in Norway (Risstad et al. 2021)<br><br>• Carpal tunnel syndrome is which pinching of the median nerve causes symptoms such as numbness, tingling and pain in the wrist, arm, or shoulder.<br>• Carpal tunnel syndrome ranges from mild to severe clinical severities.<br><br>• Surgical and non-surgical treatments exist, however the relative benefits of surgically releasing transverse ligament in the wrist is unclear.<br><br>Key outputs<br>• Based on low-certainty evidence, in patients with mild to moderate carpal tunnel syndrome surgery may be superior to splinting and combinations of non-surgical treatments<br>• For patients with severe cases, clinical guidelines, and decision tools recommend surgery as the preferred treatment<br>• Research lacks consensus on the duration of non-surgical treatment prior to proposing surgery, or whether to repeat steroid injection treatment when with insufficient effect is observed | https://www.hiqa.ie/sites/default/files/2017-01/A-Guide-to-Health-Technology-Assessment.pdf<br><br>https://www.eupati.eu/health-technology-assessment-phases-v1_en<br><br>https://www.nlm.nih.gov/nichsr/hta101/ta10103.html<br><br>Soril, L.J., Clement, F.M. and Noseworthy, T.W., 2016, November. Bioethics, health technology reassessment, and management. In Healthcare management forum (Vol. 29, No. 6, pp. 275–278). Sage CA: Los Angeles, CA: SAGE Publications.<br><br>Soril, L.J., Niven, D.J., Esmail, R., Noseworthy, T.W. and Clement, F.M. 2018. Untangling, unbundling, and moving forward: Framing health technology reassessment in the changing conceptual landscape. International Journal of Technology Assessment in Health Care, 34(2), pp. 212–217. |

| | | |
|---|---|---|
| | • Future research should address the efficacy of steroid injection versus surgery and consider the timeframe in which non-surgical patients end up receiving surgical treatment | Norburn, L. and Thomas, L., 2021. Expertise, experience, and excellence. Twenty years of patient involvement in health technology assessment at NICE: an evolving story. International Journal of Technology Assessment in Health Care, 37(1). |
| Variation study | Study of international differences in incidence and practice patterns of lower limb amputations related to peripheral arterial disease and/or diabetes mellitus showed large geographical differences in major amputation rates (Behrendt et al. 2018).<br>• Number of amputations performed per 100 000 population varied considerably – highest in Hungary and lowest in New Zealand<br>• Major amputations were more frequent in countries with lowest gross domestic product (GDP) per capita and healthcare expenditures<br>• Comparison of background factors and predictive factors | Oakes, A.H., Sen, A.P. and Segal, J.B., 2020. Understanding geographic variation in systemic overuse among the privately insured. Medical care, 58(3), pp. 257–264.<br><br>Blaser, M.J., Melby, M.K., Lock, M. and Nichter, M., 2021. Accounting for variation in and overuse of antibiotics among humans. BioEssays, 43(2), p. 2000163. |

## KEY POINTS

- Identification of low-value services must account for the inherent challenges posed by the context of the health service in question.
- Proper identification is important in order to ensure that patients receive the most appropriate and highest value care.
- Identification of low-value services relies on lists, recommendations and guidelines, use of high-quality evidence, and engagement of health professionals and the public in the process.
- Identification and measurement of overuse of low-value services are part of an interconnected process and should feed one another.

## SOURCES OF FURTHER INFORMATION

- Choosing Wisely (https://www.choosingwisely.org)
- Cochrane Collaboration (www.cochranelibrary.com)
- US Preventive Services Task Force (www.uspreventiveservicestaskforce.org)

## FURTHER READING

Balk, E.M., Earley, A., Hadar, N. et al. (2014). *Benefits and Harms of Routine Preoperative Testing: Comparative Effectiveness*. Rockville (MD): Agency for Healthcare Research and Quality. Comparative Effectiveness Review.

Behrendt, C.A., Sigvant, B., Szeberin, Z. et al. (2018). International variations in amputation practice: a VASCUNET report. *European Journal of Vascular and Endovascular Surgery* 56 (3): 391–399.

Bhatia, R.S., Bouck, Z., Ivers, N.M. et al. (2017). Electrocardiograms in low-risk patients undergoing an annual health examination. *JAMA Internal Medicine* 177 (9): 1326–1333.

Blaser, M.J., Melby, M.K., Lock, M. et al. (2021). Accounting for variation in and overuse of antibiotics among humans. *BioEssays* 43: 2000163.

Cassel, C.K. and Guest, J.A. (2012). Choosing Wisely: helping physicians and patients make smart decisions about their care. *Journal of the American Medical Association* 307: 1801–1802.

Choosing Wisely Canada. (2022). Choosing Wisely Canada Recommendations: Recommendations and Resources, by Specialty. Choosing Wisely Canada. https://choosingwiselycanada.org/recommendations (accessed September 2022).

Cliff, B.Q., Avancena, A.L., Hirth, R.A. et al. (2021). The impact of Choosing Wisely interventions on low-value medical services: a systematic review. *The Milbank Quarterly* 99: 1024–1058.

van Dulmen, S.A., Tran, N.H., Wiersma, T. et al. (2022). Identifying and prioritizing do-not-do recommendations in Dutch primary care. *BMC Prim Care* 23: 141.

Ellen, M.E., Wilson, M.G., Vélez, M. et al. (2018). Addressing overuse of health services in health systems: a critical interpretive synthesis. *Health Research Policy and Systems* 16: 1–14.

Elshaug, A.G., Bessen, T., Moss, J.R. et al. (2010). Addressing "waste" in diagnostic imaging: some implications of comparative effectiveness research. *Journal of the American College of Radiology* 7 (8): 603–613.

Guirguis-Blake, J.M., Webber, E.M., and Coppola, E.L. (2021). Screening for asymptomatic carotid artery stenosis in the general population: updated evidence report and systematic review for the US Preventive Services Task Force. *JAMA* 325 (5): 487–489.

Henrikson, N.B., Aiello Bowles, E.J., Blasi, P.R. et al. (2019). Screening for pancreatic cancer: updated evidence report and systematic review for the US Preventive Services Task Force. *JAMA* 322 (5): 445–454.

Institute of Medicine (2011). Committee on standards for developing trustworthy clinical practice guidelines. In: *Clinical Practice Guidelines we Can Trust* (ed. R. Graham et al.). Washington, DC: The National Academies Press.

Kirk, P.S., Borza, T., Caram, M.E. et al. (2019). Characterising potential bone scan overuse amongst men treated with radical prostatectomy. *BJU International* 124: 55–61.

Kirkham, K.R., Wijeysundera, D.N., Pendrith, C. et al. (2015). Preoperative testing before low-risk surgical procedures. *Canadian Medical Association Journal* 187: E349–E358.

Lee, A.L., Burge, A.T., and Holland, A.E. (2015). Airway clearance techniques for bronchiectasis. *Cochrane Database Syst Rev.* 11: CD008351.

Levinson, W., Born, K., and Wolfson, D. (2018). Choosing Wisely campaigns: a work in Progress. *Journal of the American Medical Association* 319: 1975–1976.

Moore, L., Lauzier, F., Tardif, P.-A. et al. (2019). Low-value clinical practices in injury care: a scoping review and expert consultation survey. *Journal of Trauma and Acute Care Surgery* 86: 983–993.

Mustafa, R.A., Santesso, N., Brozek, J. et al. (2013). The GRADE approach is reproducible in assessing the quality of evidence of quantitative evidence syntheses. *Journal of Clinical Epidemiology* 66: 736–742; quiz 742 e731-735.

Norburn, L. and Thomas, L. (2021). Expertise, experience, and excellence. Twenty years of patient involvement in health technology assessment at NICE: an evolving story. *International Journal of Technology Assessment in Health Care* 37.

Oakes, A.H., Sen, A.P., and Segal, J.B. (2020). Understanding geographic variation in systemic overuse among the privately insured. *Medical Care* 58: 257–264.

Padula, W.V., Berzon, R.A., Mujuru, P. et al. (2021). Comparative effectiveness research in health disparity populations. *The Science of Health Disparities Research* 359–374. http://doi.org/10.1002/9781119374855.ch21.

Postmus, D., Richard, S., Bere, N. et al. (2018). Individual trade-offs between possible benefits and risks of Cancer treatments: results from a stated preference study with patients with multiple myeloma. *The Oncologist* 23: 44–51.

Risstad, H., Hamidi, V., Espeland, A.L. et al. (2021). *Surgical Treatment of Carpal Tunnel Syndrome: A Health Technology Assessment.* Norwegian Oslo: Norwegian Institute of Public Health.

Sheridan, S.L., Sutkowi-Hemstreet, A., Barclay, C. et al. (2016). A comparative effectiveness trial of alternate formats for presenting benefits and harms information for low-value screening services: a randomized clinical trial. *JAMA Internal Medicine* 176: 31–41.

Society of Hospital Medicine (Choosing Wisely) (2022). Adult Hospital Medicine: Eleven Things Physicians and Patients Should Question. https://www.choosingwisely.org/societies/society-of-hospital-medicine-adult/ (accessed 24 April 2023).

Soril, L.J., Clement, F.M., and Noseworthy, T.W. (2016). Bioethics, health technology reassessment, and management. *Healthcare Management Forum* 275–278, SAGE Publications Sage CA: Los Angeles, CA.

Soril, L.J., Niven, D.J., Esmail, R. et al. (2018). Untangling, unbundling, and moving forward: framing health technology reassessment in the changing conceptual landscape. *International Journal of Technology Assessment in Health Care* 34: 212–217.

USPSTF. (2012). Grade Defenitions. U.S. Preventive Services Task Force. https://www.uspreventiveservicestaskforce.org/uspstf/about-uspstf/methods-and-processes/grade-definitions#july2012 (accessed September 2022).

Veloudi, P., Jones, G., and Sharman, J.E. (2017). Effectiveness of Vitamin D supplementation for cardiovascular health outcomes. *Pulse (Basel)* 4: 193–207.

Verkerk, E.W., Huisman-de Waal, G., Vermeulen, H. et al. (2018). Low-value care in nursing: a systematic assessment of clinical practice guidelines. *International Journal of Nursing Studies* 87: 34–39.

Wammes, J.J., van den Akker-van Marle, M.E., Verkerk, E.W. et al. (2016). Identifying and prioritizing lower value services from Dutch specialist guidelines and a comparison with the UK do-not-do list. *BMC Medicine* 14: 196.

# CHAPTER 7

# Measuring Low-Value Care and Choosing Your Local Priority (Phase 1)

Carole E. Aubert[1,2], Karen Born[3], Eve A. Kerr[4,5,6], Sacha Bhatia[7,8], and Eva W. Verkerk[9]

[1] Department of General Internal Medicine, Bern University Hospital, Inselspital, Bern, Switzerland
[2] Institute of Primary Health Care (BIHAM), University of Bern, Bern, Switzerland
[3] Institute for Health Policy, Management & Evaluation, University of Toronto, Toronto, Ontario, Canada
[4] Center for Clinical Management Research, Veterans Affairs Ann Arbor Healthcare System, Ann Arbor, Michigan, United States
[5] Institute for Healthcare Policy and Innovation, University of Michigan, Ann Arbor, Michigan, United States
[6] Department of Internal Medicine, University of Michigan, Ann Arbor, Michigan, United States
[7] Department of Medicine, University of Toronto, Toronto, Ontario, Canada
[8] Institute for Health System Solutions and Virtual Care, Women's College Hospital, Toronto, Ontario, Canada
[9] Department of IQ Healthcare, Radboud University Medical Center, Radboud Institute for Health Sciences, Nijmegen, The Netherlands

## CHOOSING YOUR LOCAL PRIORITY

It is not possible to de-implement all low-value care practices at the same time; you should choose local priorities to work on (Grimshaw et al. 2020). Focusing efforts on a few practices that can realistically be reduced is likely to be more effective than spreading insufficient resources across multiple practices. There are several criteria to consider when selecting your local priority. First, the low-value care practice should be present in high rates in the setting where you want to reduce it. Second, reducing the low-value care practice should improve the outcomes for patients, healthcare professionals, and/or healthcare systems in your setting. Third, there should be a possibility to address any major barriers faced by patients and healthcare professionals to ensure effectiveness. Fourth, it is helpful to have the support of a local clinical leader who can advocate for the initiative. Fifth, the intervention to reduce the low-value care practice must be feasible and adequately resourced (including employee, time, and financial resources). Sixth, initiatives to reduce low-value care often require multiple components, e.g. education, quality improvement tools, measurement, and evaluation (Cliff et al. 2021). These can be costly and time-consuming. Therefore, we should assess which components are needed, a process that we will describe in Chapter 8. This can help to assess whether the effort is 'worth it' and likely feasible before starting a de-implementation initiative (Bhatia et al. 2015) and whether the components are available, to ensure that the measure can be used (Chan et al. 2013).

## MEASURING LOW-VALUE CARE

Measuring the impact of de-implementation initiatives is crucial to provide evidence on the effectiveness of the initiative and knowledge on how to improve and spread the intervention(s). Measuring low-value care includes baseline and impact measurements.

## Baseline Measurements

Once you have defined and identified potential low-value care practice(s) to target as described in Chapter 6, you should perform key baseline measurements. These might include measuring the volume, rates, and variability of the practice(s). Volume is a common metric in healthcare to evaluate the frequency or quantity of a particular service or practice. Rates offer an indication of the frequency of the practice using a relationship to a fixed standard or unit. Variability is a common measure in healthcare quality that demonstrates differences in the use of a practice in different settings, such as healthcare professionals, regions, or populations (e.g. hospital versus ambulatory care; younger versus older patients). The assessment of volume, rates, and variability helps evaluate the magnitude of a low-value care practice in your setting. It also provides information on the targets with the most potential for improvement, as well as on the resources required to de-implement the targeted low-value care practice. Finally, it provides baseline information to estimate the potential volume reduction and financial impact of the intervention.

Often, you may have to use a proxy measure, as it is not possible to measure directly a low-value care practice (Chalmers et al. 2018). The available data may be insufficiently detailed to clearly distinguish low-value from high-value care. For example, to measure the frequency of low-value imaging for non-specific low back pain, you could use the total volume of imaging as a proxy. However, this evaluation does not account for the presence of 'red flags', indicating that imaging could be appropriate (Rao and Levin 2012; Hall et al. 2021). The assessment of imaging alone is, thus, neither a specific nor an accurate reflection of low-value care. Nevertheless, such a proxy measure, despite not being specific, might still be a helpful indicator and might be the only way to approach the measurement of a low-value care practice in some instances.

The volume, rate, and variability of a low-value care practice are often expressed as a proportion or percentage. However, this number might vary greatly depending on the denominator used: patients, population, or services (Chalmers et al. 2017).

A study showed, for example, that, from the patients' perspective, 16.2% of patients with syncope had an unnecessary carotid ultrasound. From the population perspective, 0.7% of the population had both syncope and a carotid ultrasound. And from a service perspective, 6.5% of the patients who received a carotid ultrasound had syncope. Therefore, it is very important to carefully observe numerator and denominator especially when comparing low-value care rates. The patient perspective is used most often and is most likely to show a significant reduction.

## ESTIMATING IMPROVEMENT POTENTIAL

Reducing low-value care is an important quality priority for many organisations but can be resource intensive and time-consuming. It is, therefore, important to focus de-implementation efforts on low-value care practices where reduction is likely to improve outcomes or reduce inappropriate costs. Therefore, you should estimate the potential for outcome improvement and for the reduction of inappropriate costs in your setting before starting to develop or implement any intervention. In addition to measuring current volume of low-value care, this can include various assessments, such as patient-relevant outcomes and experiences (PROMs and PREMs), effects on healthcare professional experiences, effects on the healthcare systems and on the healthcare policy, as well as employee and material costs (Berwick and Hackbarth 2012; Shrank et al. 2019; Hood and Weinberger 2012; Maratt et al. 2019; Norton and Chambers 2020). These assessments are specific to each low-value care practice.

## EVALUATING DE-IMPLEMENTATION EFFECTS

This section describes measurements that you can use to assess the effect of your de-implementation initiative. Other aspects of the evaluation, such as the study design and process evaluation, are discussed in Chapter 10. The success of your initiatives to reduce low-value care depends on their short-, medium-, and long-term effects on the patients and the healthcare professionals. It is crucial that the outcome measures you chose reflect not only the type of action, but also the time horizon in which those outcomes should be achieved (Norton and Chambers 2020). The long-term effects of an initiative can help to predict whether the effects will be sustained. Table 7.1 describes an overview of potential measure types with examples (Aubert et al. 2020; Maratt et al. 2019).

**TABLE 7.1** De-implementation measures.

| Measure type | Examples |
| --- | --- |
| Appropriateness (over-, under-, misuse) | Overuse: proportion of patients with low back pain without 'red flags' who receive low back imaging <br> Underuse: Rates of C-section in high-risk births |
| | Misuse: Proportion of patients receiving benzodiazepines for sleep problems during hospitalisation |
| Utilisation/ordering | Percent of repeated lab test |
| Outcomes | Readmissions |
| Patient-reported outcome measures | Quality of life scale |
| Patient-reported experience measures | Satisfaction with care |
| Patient preferences | Patient preference for shared decision-making |
| Provider-reported experience | Self-reported comfort level of staff with intervention |
| Patient-provider interaction | Shared Decision Making Process Scale |
| Value (outcome/cost) | Cost-effectiveness |
| Cost | In-hospital costs |

Source: Adapted from Maratt et al. 2019.

Bhatia et al. (2015) highlighted three important types of impact of initiatives to reduce low-value care:

- Changes in healthcare professional attitudes and awareness regarding the low-value care practice.
- Changes in healthcare professional behaviours such as communication with patients and prescribing the low-value care practice.
- Patients' perceptions and outcomes regarding the low-value care practice.

Their framework provides an integrative and comprehensive approach to the measurement of interventions to reduce low-value care (Bhatia et al. 2015). We illustrate this approach in Box 7.1 using the example of imaging for low back pain.

## Box 7.1   Comprehensive Approach: Example of Imaging for Low Back Pain

'Do not do imaging for low back pain within the first six weeks, unless red flags are present' is a *Choosing Wisely* recommendation across a number of country campaigns (Rao and Levin 2012; Hall et al. 2021). The integrated approach of measurement comprises different interrelated steps. Depending on the type of low-value care and improvement initiative, not all steps are required or appropriate. First, administrative data can be used to provide information on variability of use of imaging for low back pain, which can help create awareness of the problem amongst healthcare professionals. Second, surveys and interviews of healthcare professionals can be used to assess the barriers and facilitators to de-implementation, which can support the design of the intervention (as described in Chapters 8 and 9). Third, patient surveys and interviews about their perceptions of the low-value practice and their care can be used to ensure that the de-implementation leads to more patient-centred care. They can also help to monitor the level of low back pain experienced by the patients and any unintended consequences. Fourth, clinical data are useful to monitor for unintended consequences, such as the underuse of low back imaging when it is actually indicated, i.e. when a 'red flag' is present, or substitution for an alternative low-value practice. Finally, detailed clinical data also allow one to determine rates of low back imaging, distinguishing between low-value (i.e. imaging without 'red flags that is inappropriate') and high-value (i.e. imaging with 'red flags that is appropriate') care. These measurements provide feedback to healthcare professionals, which can in return act as motivational factors to improve practices. Furthermore, they allow the identification of outliers and taking actions to address what drives their behaviour.

Several organisations, including the Agency for Healthcare Research and Quality in the United States (https://quality indicators.ahrq.gov) and the National Institute for Health and Care Excellence in the United Kingdom (www.nice.org.uk/standards-and-indicators), have already developed measures (also called performance indicators) that can be applied or adapted for the purpose of initiatives to reduce low-value care. In addition, the United States' Lown Institute (https://lown hospitalsindex.org) has combined several measures to rank hospitals based on their level of avoiding overuse and delivering cost-efficient care. It is worthwhile checking whether there is already a measure in use for the low-value care practice that you want to address.

## MEASURING UNINTENDED CONSEQUENCES

Initiatives to reduce low-value care practices can have unintended consequences, which should be carefully monitored (Baker et al. 2013; Mathias and Baker 2013; Baker and Qaseem 2011; Colla et al. 2017; Maratt et al. 2019; Norton and

Chambers 2020). What are potential unintended consequences? First, reducing low-value care can lead to underuse of the service being intervened upon or of related high-value care services. For example, recommending against systematically measuring vitamin D levels in older adults may lead to not measuring vitamin D when it would actually be indicated e.g. in patients with osteoporosis. Second, reducing low-value care may lead to a substitution for an alternative low-value practice. For example, reducing the use of benzodiazepines can lead to inappropriate prescribing of sedative antidepressants. Third, reducing low-value care may affect patient and healthcare professional experience and their interaction e.g. patient dissatisfaction, and disruption in healthcare professional–patient relationship (Bhatia et al. 2015). Fourth, reducing low-value care may lead to care location shift or increased costs. For example, a patient denied antibiotics by their outpatient healthcare professional for a likely viral infection might go to the emergency room for a second advice. Fifth, harmful consequences may happen. For example, deprescribing benzodiazepines can lead to withdrawal symptoms. Therefore, it is important to recognise potential unintended consequences. Additional examples of measures of unintended consequences are provided in Table 7.2.

## MEASUREMENT METHODS AND DATA SOURCE

You can measure outcomes using a variety of methods including direct observations, surveys, focus groups, interviews, administrative databases, electronic health records, chart data, and prospective data collection. Each method and data source presents advantages and disadvantages, as explained in Table 7.3. The type of measurement method depends on the target population and outcomes. Healthcare professionals' attitudes and awareness are typically evaluated through surveys, focus groups, or interviews. How to perform these will be described in more detail in Chapter 8. Healthcare professionals' behaviours are best evaluated using administrative, electronic health record, or chart data.

**TABLE 7.2**   Measures of unintended consequences.

| Measure of unintended consequences type | Examples |
|---|---|
| Substitution for alternative low-value practice | Proportion of patients with benzodiazepine deprescribing who are prescribed another sedative medication |
| Underuse of the service being intervened upon/of related practices | Proportion of patients with pneumonia and indication for antibiotic who do not receive antibiotic |
| Patient-reported experience | Anxiety |
| Provider-reported experience | Fear of missing a diagnosis |
| Patient-provider interaction | Patient-Doctor Interaction Scale |
| Patient selection | Care provision according to insurance status |
| Care location shift | Visit of a specialist for the same reason |
| Harm (outcome) | Mortality |
| Reimbursement | Additional costs for the patients (e.g. if service not any more reimbursed) |

Source: Adapted from Maratt et al. 2019.

Finally, patients' perceptions and outcomes, such as their engagement and acceptance of the initiatives, are usually evaluated through surveys or interviews. They consist of patient-reported experience measures (PREMs) and patient-reported outcomes measures (PROMs). Additional patient outcomes, such as the adverse effects of low-value care, are best evaluated using administrative, electronic health record, or chart data. The use of existing data is usually preferable, because it is less resource intensive and leverages data already present in a healthcare system or practice. However, existing data are not always accurate or available.

**TABLE 7.3** Advantages and disadvantages of measurement tools according to measurement area.

| Measurement tool | Measurement area | |
|---|---|---|
| | Advantages | Disadvantages |
| *Healthcare professional attitudes and awareness* | | |
| Surveys | Cheap, high number, possible resample, comparisons across settings | Potentially low response rates, lack of in-depth information |
| Focus groups / Interviews | More detailed information, identification of factors not pre-identified by researchers | Expensive and time-consuming |
| *Healthcare professional behaviours* | | |
| Observation | Assessment of actual behaviour in clinical practice, detailed information | Risk of influencing behaviour by presence, time-consuming |
| Administrative databases | Population- and patient-level data, information on regional variability/ comparisons across settings, easy to reassess over time, monitoring of underuse as unintended consequence | Lack of clinical details limits specificity and preclude measuring more complex recommendations |
| Electronic health record/ chart data | More clinical data than administrative data, easy to reassess over time, monitoring of underuse as unintended consequence | Some information gaps Often single-centre limited (different systems) Time and resource consuming |

(Continued)

**TABLE 7.3** (Continued)

| | Measurement area | |
|---|---|---|
| Measurement tool | Advantages | Disadvantages |
| Patient perceptions and outcomes | | |
| Survey assessing PROMs/PREMs | Standardised data collection, monitoring for unintended consequences, comparable across settings, validated tools | No questions specifically on low-value care, mediating role of cognitive bias |

Abbreviations: PREM: patient-reported experience measure; PROM: patient-reported outcome measure.
Source: Adapted from Bhatia et al. 2015.

## SETTING SPECIFIC, MEASURABLE, ACHIEVABLE, RELEVANT, AND TIME-BOUND (SMART) TARGETS

When planning a de-implementation initiative, you should define a 'SMART' target (Doran 1981). It can help checking whether your planned initiative will be feasible. For example, to reduce benzodiazepine prescribing, a non-SMART target could be 'to stop benzodiazepines'. A SMART target could be 'to reduce, within five years, by 10%, new benzodiazepine prescriptions in older adults during hospitalisation, addressing both patient, and health-care professional barriers'. Table 7.4 explains why the first target is not SMART and the second target is SMART.

## PROVIDING DATA AND FEEDBACK TO STAKEHOLDERS

If you have collected outcome measures, you can provide data and feedback to stakeholders. This is key to increase their aware-ness of the current state of low-value care, to motivate them to

**TABLE 7.4**   Examples of non-SMART and SMART targets.

| Acronym | Non-SMART target: 'To stop benzodiazepines' | SMART target: "To reduce, within five years, by 10%, new benzodiazepine prescriptions in older adults during hospitalisation, addressing both patient, and healthcare professional barriers. |
|---|---|---|
| **S**pecific | Settings/populations not defined | Population/setting/ prescription types (=new) defined |
| **M**easurable | Comparison/data source not defined | We can measure percentage of prescriptions before and after the initiative |
| **A**chievable | Too broad target, complete stop targeted, unclear if barriers addressed or funding provided | Barriers considered |
| **R**ealistic | | 10% reduction (not complete cessation) |
| **T**ime-bound | Time period not described | Duration specified |

(further) accept and engage in improvement efforts, and to validate the (ongoing) efforts (Bhatia et al. 2015). When discussing data with stakeholders, you can take the opportunity to also identify barriers, facilitators, and potential interventions. Methods for this assessment are described in Chapter 8. You can provide oral and written feedback in different ways, including mails, audits, or open discussions. The use of audit and feedback has notably been used with some success to reduce the inappropriate use of several low-value services such as antibiotics (Daneman et al. 2021; Schwartz et al. 2021). More information on interventions and other examples of audit and feedback are described in Chapters 8 and 9.

## KEY POINTS

- The volume, rates, and variability of low-value care practices and the potential of outcome improvement should be measured when choosing a local priority for a de-implementation initiative and to have a baseline for assessing the effectiveness of your initiative.
- You can evaluate the impact of initiatives on the short, medium, and long term, in several measurement areas, including healthcare professional attitudes, awareness, and behaviours, as well as patient perceptions.
- Initiatives to reduce low-value care can have unintended consequences, such as increasing underuse of care, which should be carefully monitored and assessed.
- Providing feedback to stakeholders can help to motivate them in their efforts to reduce low-value care.
- It is important to set a SMART target to check the feasibility of the planned intervention.

## REFERENCES

Agency for Healthcare Research and Quality. Quality indicators. https://qualityindicators.ahrq.gov (accessed 28 September 2022).

Aubert, C.E., Kerr, E.A., Maratt, J.K. et al. (2020). Outcome measures for interventions to reduce inappropriate chronic drugs: a narrative review. *Journal of the American Geriatrics Society* 68: 2390–2398.

Baker, D.W. and Qaseem, A. (2011). Evidence-based performance measures: preventing unintended consequences of quality measurement. *Annals of Internal Medicine* 155: 638–640.

Baker, D.W., Qaseem, A., Reynolds, P.P. et al. (2013). Design and use of performance measures to decrease low-value services and achieve cost-conscious care. *Annals of Internal Medicine* 158: 55–59.

Berwick, D.M. and Hackbarth, A.D. (2012). Eliminating waste in US health care. *JAMA* 307: 1513–1516.

Bhatia, R.S., Levinson, W., Shortt, S. et al. (2015). Measuring the effect of Choosing Wisely: an integrated framework to assess campaign impact on low-value care. *BMJ Quality and Safety* 24: 523–531.

Chalmers, K., Pearson, S.A., and Elshaug, A.G. (2017). Quantifying low-value care: a patient-centric versus service-centric lens. *BMJ Quality and Safety* 26: 855–858.

Chalmers, K., Badgery-Parker, T., Pearson, S.A. et al. (2018). Developing indicators for measuring low-value care: mapping Choosing Wisely recommendations to hospital data. *BMC Research Notes* 11: 163.

Chan, K.S., Chang, E., Nassery, N. et al. (2013). The state of overuse measurement: a critical review. *Medical Care Research and Review* 70: 473–496.

Cliff, B.Q., Avanceña, A.L.V., Hirth, R.A. et al. (2021). The impact of Choosing Wisely interventions on low-value medical services: a systematic review. *The Milbank Quarterly* 99: 1024–1058.

Colla, C.H., Mainor, A.J., Hargreaves, C. et al. (2017). Interventions aimed at reducing use of low-value health services: a systematic review. *Medical Care Research and Review* 74: 507–550.

Daneman, N., Lee, S.M., Bai, H. et al. (2021). Population-wide peer comparison audit and feedback to reduce antibiotic initiation and duration in long-term care facilities with embedded randomized controlled trial. *Clinical Infectious Diseases* 73: e1296–e1304.

Doran, G.T. (1981). There's a S.M.A.R.T. way to write management's goals and objectives. *Management Review* 70 (11): 35–36.

Grimshaw, J.M., Patey, A.M., Kirkham, K.R. et al. (2020). De-implementing wisely: developing the evidence base to reduce low-value care. *BMJ Quality and Safety* 29: 409–417.

Hall, A.M., Aubrey-Bassler, K., Thorne, B. et al. (2021). Do not routinely offer imaging for uncomplicated low back pain. *BMJ* 372: n291.

Hood, V.L. and Weinberger, S.E. (2012). High value, cost-conscious care: an international imperative. *European Journal of Internal Medicine* 23: 495–498.

Maratt, J.K., Kerr, E.A., Klamerus, M.L. et al. (2019). Measures used to assess the impact of interventions to reduce low-value care: a systematic review. *Journal of General Internal Medicine* 34: 1857–1864.

Mathias, J.S. and Baker, D.W. (2013). Developing quality measures to address overuse. *JAMA* 309: 1897–1898.

National Institute for Health and Care Excellence. Standards and Indicators. www.nice.org.uk/standards-and-indicators. (accessed 28 September 2022).

Norton, W.E. and Chambers, D.A. (2020). Unpacking the complexities of de-implementing inappropriate health interventions. *Implementation Science* 15: 2.

Rao, V.M. and Levin, D.C. (2012). The overuse of diagnostic imaging and the Choosing Wisely initiative. *Annals of Internal Medicine* 157: 574–576.

Saini, V., Brownlee, S., Gopinath, V. et al. (2021). *Methodology of the Lown Institute Hospitals Index for Social Responsibility* (ed. https://lownhospitalsindex.org). Needham, MA: The Lown Institute.

Schwartz, K.L., Ivers, N., Langford, B.J. et al. (2021). Effect of antibiotic-prescribing feedback to high-volume primary care physicians on number of antibiotic prescriptions: a randomized clinical trial. *JAMA Internal Medicine* 181: 1165–1173.

Shrank, W.H., Rogstad, T.L., and Parekh, N. (2019). Waste in the US Health Care System: estimated costs and potential for savings. *JAMA* 322: 1501–1509.

# CHAPTER 8

# Identifying Target Behaviours and Potential Barriers to Change (Phase 2a)

Andrea M. Patey[1,2,3], Nicola McCleary[1,2,3,4],
Justin Presseau[1,2,3], Tijn Kool[5], Simone van Dulmen[5],
and Jeremy M. Grimshaw[1,2,3,6]

[1] Centre for Implementation Research, Ottawa Hospital
Research Institute, Ottawa, Ontario, Canada
[2] School of Epidemiology and Public Health, University of
Ottawa, Ottawa, Ontario, Canada
[3] Clinical Epidemiology Program, Ottawa Hospital Research
Institute, Ottawa, Ontario, Canada
[4] Eastern Ontario Regional Laboratory Association, Ottawa,
Ontario, Canada
[5] Department of IQ Healthcare, Radboud University Medical
Center, Radboud Institute for Health Sciences, Nijmegen,
The Netherlands
[6] Department of Medicine, University of Ottawa, Ottawa,
Ontario, Canada

*How to Reduce Overuse in Healthcare: A Practical Guide*, First Edition.
Edited by Tijn Kool, Andrea M. Patey, Simone van Dulmen, and Jeremy M. Grimshaw.
© 2024 John Wiley & Sons Ltd. Published 2024 by John Wiley & Sons Ltd.

## THE IMPORTANCE OF FULLY UNDERSTANDING THE PROBLEM

Chapter 2 outlines how overuse is driven by provider and patient factors as well as organisation and system factors. In Chapter 3, potential reasons for overuse are mentioned and how things may be behaviourally driven. Often at this point, people think, 'That's it, we know what the reasons are for overuse! Let us fix it!' and move right to brainstorming solutions without fully understanding the problem in their context or environment. Colloquially, the process has been coined the 'ISLAGIATT principle', where the justification for the proposed solution was that 'it seemed like a good idea at the time' (Colquhoun et al. 2013). However, it is important to know the specific drivers of current behaviour and barriers to desired behaviours in your setting because some of the factors identified in Chapters 2 and 3 may be more relevant to your specific setting than others. The identification of solutions without fully understanding the problem may lead to interventions being introduced that do not actually address the problem. Interventions consume valuable resources in the context of healthcare systems, where resources are finite. Taking time to identify and address the key barriers helps ensure that resources are invested in interventions that are tailor-made and fit-for-purpose, have greater probability of success, and helps ensure that critical resources are not wasted.

Phase 2 of the de-implementing wisely framework (see Chapter 4) focuses on the identification of barriers and enablers to implementing recommendations and potential interventions to overcome these. In this chapter, we focus on identifying barriers and enablers. Chapter 9 will guide readers through the process of identifying potential interventions to overcome identified barriers.

## GETTING STARTED

It may be difficult to know where to start when trying to think of an intervention to reduce low-value care. One approach is to ask oneself four questions (French et al. 2012):

1. Who needs to do what, differently?
2. Using a theoretical framework, which barriers and enablers need to be addressed?
3. Which intervention components could overcome the modifiable barriers and enhance the enablers?
4. How can behaviour change be measured and understood?

By going through the process of trying to answer these four questions, you can clearly identify the problem (who needs to do what, differently?), better assess the problem (using a theoretical framework, which barriers and enablers need to be addressed?), form possible solutions to the problem (which intervention components could overcome the modifiable barriers and enhance the enablers?), and outline how we will evaluate our solution to determine whether it fixed the problem (how can behaviour change be measured and understood?) (French et al. 2012). This chapter guides readers through the first two questions and suggests tools one could use to help clearly identify and assess the overuse problem. The subsequent chapters focus on designing interventions (see Chapter 9) and evaluation of those interventions (see Chapter 10).

## IDENTIFYING WHO NEEDS TO DO WHAT DIFFERENTLY

De-implementation of low-value care may require different people to do different things at different times in different settings. Wang et al. (2018) identify four different types of de-implementation: partial reversal, complete reversal, related replacement, and unrelated replacement. Partial reversal implies that a clinical practice behaviour should be stopped for a sub-group of the patient population based on new evidence. In the United States, breast cancer screening used to be recommended for women over 40; the 2015 guidelines recommend that women over 45 years of age should be screened (Oeffinger et al. 2015). Complete reversal implies that the clinical practice behaviour should be stopped entirely. In Canada, for example, chest X-rays are no longer recommended for individuals undergoing cataract surgery (Dobson et al. 2021). Replacement, such as using intermittent auscultation instead of continuous foetal monitoring for people in labour (Patey et al. 2017), and unrelated replacement, such as using a viral prescription pad instead of prescribing antibiotics for people with respiratory tract infections (Lee et al. 2020), require the cessation or reduction of a low-value care using a potential strategy (behaviour substitution) (Michie et al. 2013). How that happens, whether using behaviour substitution or other techniques, will be discussed in Chapter 9.

These four examples demonstrate how reducing low-value care can require different types of clinical behaviour change at the point of interaction with the patient. But other people in the health system may also have to change the way they work to ensure that the low-value care is de-implemented. For example, reducing low-value pre-operative tests for low-risk patients may require changes to policies and procedures at the healthcare organisation level (as well as healthcare professional behaviour change). At the organisational level, heads of department (surgery, anaesthesiology, and medicine) may need to meet to write a hospital policy that guides hospital staff to appropriate preoperative test ordering. Something that appears as simple as reducing low-value preoperative tests requires a myriad of different people at different times to do different things. The importance of detailed behaviour specification can help to identify all the key people and what they do as well as to clarify evidence–practice gaps and who needs to be doing what differently.

## USING THE ACTION, ACTOR, CONTEXT, TARGET, TIME (AACTT) FRAMEWORK

The 'AACTT' framework (Actor [which individual should do this], Action [the observable act], Context [where], Target [from whom is the action being performed; often the patient], Time [when] [Presseau et al. 2019]) specifies behaviours in healthcare contexts using common elements that can be used for consistent description and monitoring of clinical behaviours. Box 8.1 provides an example of using the AACTT to specify a single-actor healthcare behaviour.

**Box 8.1   Use of the AACTT Framework to Specify 'Not Ordering Routine Preoperative Tests for Low-Risk Surgical Procedures' (Single Actor)**

| AACTT | Single actor and single action |
| --- | --- |
| **ACTION** (Specify the BEHAVIOUR that needs to change in terms that can be observed or measured) | **Ordering preoperative tests like electrocardiographs and chest X-rays** |
| **ACTOR** (Specify the PERSON who do(es) or could do the action) | **Anaesthesiologists** |
| **CONTEXT** (Specify the physical location, emotional context, or social setting IN WHICH the action is performed) | **In the consultation room** |
| **TARGET** (Specify the person/ people FOR WHOM the action is performed) | **Asymptomatic patients undergoing low-risk surgical procedure** |
| **TIME** (Specify WHEN the action needs to be performed – time, date, and frequency) | **During preoperative assessment** |

The AACTT framework can also be used to describe the sequence of multiple behaviours of multiple actors engaging in their own action at different levels of the organisation required to enact change (Presseau et al. 2019). The AACTT framework helps to unpack the complexity and clarify which stakeholders need to enact specific behaviours in healthcare settings, rather than making assumptions about such a sequence of behaviours or describing them as independent factors. Box 8.2 provides an example of specifying behaviours by multiple actors using the AACTT principle. One or all these behaviours could be the focus of a de-implementation intervention, depending on resources available.

Box 8.2 Use of the AACTT Framework to Specify Behaviours Involved in 'Not Ordering Routine Preoperative Tests for Low-Risk Surgical Procedures' (Multiple-Actor Example)

| AACTT | Multiple actors and multiple behaviours | | |
|---|---|---|---|
| ACTION (Specify the BEHAVIOUR that needs to change it term that can be observed or measured) | Ordering preoperative tests like electrocardiographs and Chest x-rays | Confirming appropriate test ordering | Writing hospital policy |
| ACTOR (Specify the PERSON who do(es) or could do the action) | Anaesthesiologists | Preoperative Nurse | Chiefs/department heads of Anaesthesia and Surgery |
| CONTEXT (Specify the physical location, emotional context, or social setting IN WHICH the action is performed) | In the consultation room | In the consultation room | Staff meeting |
| TARGET (Specify the person/people FOR WHOM the action is performed) | Asymptomatic patients undergoing low-risk surgical procedure | Anaesthesiologist | Anaesthesiologist |
| TIME (Specify WHEN the action needs to be performed – time, date, and frequency) | During preoperative assessment | During Preoperative assessment | Initial set-up |

By clearly specifying the low-value care that needs to stop, you promote clarity to others regarding expectations for the project and what will be the focus, as well as helping to identify what should be measured when evaluating de-implementation change projects, as discussed in Chapter 10.

## IDENTIFYING DRIVERS OF CURRENT BEHAVIOUR AND BARRIERS AND ENABLERS TO CHANGING BEHAVIOUR

De-implementation of low-value care needs key actors to change their behaviour. The AACTT frameworks helps identify which key actors in your context may need to change their behaviour. The next key step involves identifying the drivers of current behaviour and barriers and enablers to changing behaviour; this usually involves conducting surveys or focus groups with a small number of actors in your setting. You may also need to observe people in the clinic to see what happens at the point of care with patients. However, observational studies may be time-consuming; the feasibility to do this may be limited.

Applying a behavioural approach can be beneficial to your investigation of the drivers of current behaviour and barriers and enablers to changing it. Behavioural science theories provide a valuable foundation from which to understand the factors that may explain and influence why healthcare providers face challenges with de-implementing low-value care (Eccles et al. 2007; Grimshaw et al. 2011). Behavioural theories can also help you understand the mediators (mechanisms) and moderators (effect modifiers) between behavioural influences and interventions in the environments (policy, system, organisation, or team) (Sniehotta et al. 2017) in which healthcare professionals work. Applying a theory-driven approach helps build on what we already know about determinants of behaviour and how to change behaviour.

There are many behavioural theories that you could use to investigate the factors that influence clinical behaviours

(Davis et al. 2014). Selecting a theory to apply in your setting can feel daunting. One of the tools from behavioural sciences designed to make theories more accessible to those working in de-implementation is the TDF (Atkins et al. 2017). The TDF is a comprehensive framework that examines individual-, organisational-, and structural-level barriers and enablers to healthcare provider behaviours. The TDF includes 14 theoretical construct 'domains' to describe modifiable factors that can influence healthcare professional behaviour (Cane et al. 2012). These domains are described in Table 8.1 (Grimshaw et al. 2020). The TDF helps understand individual, sociocultural, and environmental influences on behaviour in specific contexts (Prothero et al. 2021).

**TABLE 8.1** Theoretical Domains Framework domains and their explanations.

| Domain | Description |
|---|---|
| Knowledge | Existing procedural knowledge, knowledge about guidelines, knowledge about evidence, and how those influences what the participants do |
| Skills | Competence and ability about the procedural techniques required to perform the behaviour |
| Social/professional role and identity | Boundaries between professional groups (i.e. is the behaviour something the participant is supposed to do or someone else's role?) |
| Beliefs about capabilities | Perceptions about competence and confidence in doing the behaviour and how that influences their behaviour |
| Optimism | Whether the participant's optimism or pessimism about the behaviour influences what they do |
| Beliefs about consequences | Perceptions about outcomes, advantages, and disadvantages of performing the behaviour and how those influences whether they perform the behaviour |

**TABLE 8.1** (Continued)

| Domain | Description |
| --- | --- |
| Reinforcement | Previous experiences that have influenced whether or not the behaviour is performed |
| Intention | A conscious decision to perform a behaviour or a resolve to act in a certain way |
| Goals | Priorities, importance, and commitment to a certain course of actions or behaviours |
| Memory, attention, and decision processes | Attention control, decision-making, memory (i.e. is the target behaviour problematic because people simply forget?) |
| Environmental context and resources | How factors related to the setting in which the behaviour is performed (e.g. people, organisational, cultural, political, physical, and financial factors) influence the behaviour |
| Social influences | External influence from people or groups to perform or not perform the behaviour How the views of colleagues, other professions, patients and families, and doing what you are told, influence the behaviour |
| Emotion | How feelings or affect (positive or negative) may influence the behaviour |
| Behavioural regulation | Ways of doing things that relate to pursuing and achieving desired goals, standards, or targets Strategies the participants have in place to help them perform the behaviour Strategies the participants would like to have in place to help them |

Source: Grimshaw et al. 2020/BMJ Publishing Group Ltd.

A guide has been developed to support using this framework (Atkins et al. 2017). If you want to investigate why healthcare professionals in your own organisation are providing low-value care, you might check these categories and analyse in which degree they play a role. The TDF has been used to investigate factors influencing a broad range of healthcare providers behaviours that require de-implementation, including routine ordering of preoperative tests, managing acute low back pain without ordering an X-ray, prescribing errors, and transfusing red blood cells (Atkins et al. 2017).

## COLLECTING DATA

There are several ways to collect data related to the drivers of behaviour and barriers and enablers to behaviour change, including interviews with healthcare providers, focus groups, and surveys. These options are somewhat formal means of data collection typically intended for a research or quality improvement projects and depending on your capacity and resources may not be feasible with your team and in your setting. However, the TDF can be used to guide discussions within the teams in a less formal manner to identify influencing factors. There are advantages and disadvantages to using any of these methods, and they need to be weighed equally when deciding what data collection method(s) you plan to use. Additionally, depending on resources available, you can use one or a combination of these methods.

### Interviews

Interviews are commonly used when investigating factors that influence clinical behaviours (Atkins et al. 2017). An example of interview guide using the TDF can be found in the appendix at the end of this chapter. A TDF series published in *Implementation Science* in 2012 contains several example interview guides (https://www.biomedcentral.com/collections/tdf) that you can access to start drafting your guide. Conducting these interviews with the healthcare providers directly involved in the delivery of the low-value care provides an opportunity to ask in-depth questions about their experiences in trying to stop the low-value care, potentially in more detail than the other two methods. Box 8.3 provides an example of an interview study. However, interviewing one-on-one usually requires time and resources, as well as ensures that the interviewer is skilled and trained in conducting interviews. The more practice you get in conducting the interviews, the better and richer the data will be. It is recommended that a minimum of 10 interviews be conducted for initial data analysis, followed by three additional interviews until no new ideas are identified (Francis et al. 2010). In small projects, it may be more feasible to have informal talks with the key healthcare providers rather than interviews, but the data should still be collected using structured methods.

---

### Box 8.3  Example of Interview Study Using TDF to Investigate Barriers to Reducing Low-Value Care

Routine preoperative tests are ordered by anaesthesiologists and surgeons for healthy patients undergoing low-risk surgery. The TDF was used to explore anaesthesiologists' and surgeons' perceptions of ordering routine tests for healthy patients undergoing low-risk surgery. Sixteen clinicians (eleven anaesthesiologists and five surgeons) throughout Ontario, Canada were interviewed using the TDF to identify factors influencing preoperative test ordering practices. Content analysis of physicians' statements into the relevant theoretical domains was performed. Specific beliefs were identified by grouping similar utterances of the interview participants. Relevant domains were identified by noting the frequencies of the beliefs reported, presence of conflicting beliefs, and perceived influence on the performance of the behaviour under investigation.

Seven domains were identified as likely relevant to changing clinicians' behaviour about pre-operative test ordering for anaesthesia management. Key themes within these domains include conflicting comments about who was responsible for the test ordering (Social/professional role and identity), inability to cancel tests ordered by fellow physicians (Beliefs about capabilities and Social influences), and the problem with tests being completed before the anaesthesiologists see the patient (Beliefs about capabilities and Environmental context and resources). Tests were often ordered by an anaesthesiologist based on who may be the attending anaesthesiologist on the day of surgery, while surgeons ordered tests they thought anaesthesiologists may need (Social influences). There were also conflicting comments about the potential consequences associated with reducing testing, from negative (delay or cancel patients' surgeries), to indifference (little or no change in patient outcomes), to positive (save money, avoid unnecessary investigations) (Beliefs about consequences). Further, while most agreed that they are motivated to reduce ordering unnecessary tests (Motivation and goals), there was still a report of a gap between their motivation and practice (Behavioural regulation).

*Source*: Adapted from Patey et al. 2012.

## Focus Groups

Focus groups can typically be a more efficient means of data collection than individual interviews because of the time it takes to do the individual interviews. Additionally, focus groups also allow for the interactions between group members, which may identify influencing factors to de-implementing low-value care that might not have been identified in individual interviews. However, it may be difficult to coordinate a group of healthcare professionals to meet at a set time. You may want to take advantage of existing team meetings, such as monthly rounds, or departmental meetings to connect with the key healthcare providers. Ideally, you should involve 8–10 participants in your focus group. As facilitator, you would guide the participants through the discussion, ensuring that everyone was provided the opportunity to voice their opinions about the factors that influence their practice behaviour. You may also want to consider having a person take notes or, if possible, to record the focus group so that you can capture non-verbal agreement or disagreements that may be missed during the discussion. Because healthcare contexts are often hierarchical, it may be advisable to have separate focus groups for those in different roles to encourage openness in responding. Box 8.4 provides an example of a study using focus groups for data collection.

---

**Box 8.4   Example of Focus Group Study Using TDF to Investigate Barriers to Reducing Low-Value Care**

The TDF was used to explore the beliefs of chiropractors in an American Provider Network and two Canadian provinces about their adherence to evidence-based recommendations for spine radiography for uncomplicated back pain. The primary objective of the study was to identify chiropractors' beliefs about managing uncomplicated back pain without X-rays and to explore barriers and facilitators to implementing evidence-based recommendations on lumbar spine X-rays. Six focus groups exploring beliefs about managing back pain without X-rays were conducted with a purposive sample. Focus groups were digitally recorded, transcribed verbatim, and analysed by two independent assessors using thematic content analysis based on the TDF.

Key themes within five domains included conflicting comments about the potential consequences of not ordering X-rays (risk of missing a pathology, avoiding adverse treatment effects, risks of litigation, determining the treatment plan, and using

X-ray-driven techniques contrasted with perceived benefits of minimising patient radiation exposure and reducing costs; beliefs about consequences); beliefs regarding professional autonomy, professional credibility, lack of standardisation, and agreement with guidelines widely varied (Social/professional role and identity); the influence of formal training, colleagues, and patients also appeared to be important factors (Social influences); conflicting comments regarding levels of confidence and comfort in managing patients without X-rays (Belief about capabilities); and guideline awareness and agreements (Knowledge).

*Source*: Adapted from Bussières et al. 2012.

## Surveys

Surveys or questionnaires are less commonly means of data collection but still are a useful tool to reach large numbers of individuals at relatively low costs. Surveys can also be helpful since they require less time commitment from those who are asking the questions. However, it will be more difficult to get a rich understanding of the barriers and facilitators. It is important that the questionnaire is well-designed: questions should be clear and direct and cover all relevant domains of the TDF. You may not need to include questions from all domains if there is existing, strong evidence to focus on specific domains such as qualitative studies that have already reported on barriers to change. Box 8.5 provides an example of a survey from the Canadian Using Blood Wisely initiative based on a TDF interview study conducted by Islam et al. (2012).

## Box 8.5 Example of Survey Using the Theoretical Domains Framework to Identify Barriers to De-Implementing Unnecessary Blood Transfusion

**Using Blood Wisely: Planning Survey**

Choosing Wisely Canada

Below is a quick planning survey that will help you determine what interventions may best suit your hospital. Take the time to sit down with your team to work through this survey. Team members may include: physicians, nurses, blood bank technologists, quality team members, department heads, senior leadership, project management and communications staff.

Answer the questions below. You may find that different members of the team may answer the survey differently—that's ok! The idea is to identify areas for improvement and to help direct your team to the right intervention. Once you have completed the survey, you can review your answers and suggested interventions.

**Hospital Name:**

**Contact Name:**

**Contact Email:**

**Date:**

| | | 1 Strongly Disagree | 2 Disagree | 3 Neutral | 4 Agree | 5 Strongly Agree |
|---|---|---|---|---|---|---|
| 1 | Our team knows what the guidelines say about prescribing one unit at a time and using restrictive transfusion thresholds for stable inpatients. | ○ | ○ | ○ | ○ | ○ |
| 2 | Our team fully agrees with guidelines for prescribing one unit at a time and using restrictive transfusion thresholds for stable inpatients. | ○ | ○ | ○ | ○ | ○ |
| 3 | Our team has previously encountered problems when trying to ensure that we prescribe one unit at a time and use restrictive transfusion thresholds for stable inpatients. | ○ | ○ | ○ | ○ | ○ |
| 4 | Our team finds it difficult to question our colleagues about transfusion orders that are outside of guidelines. | ○ | ○ | ○ | ○ | ○ |

| | | 1 Strongly Disagree | 2 Disagree | 3 Neutral | 4 Agree | 5 Strongly Agree |
|---|---|---|---|---|---|---|
| 5 | Other staff (prescribers, colleagues, other team members) don't seem to prescribe one unit at a time and use restrictive transfusion thresholds. | ○ | ○ | ○ | ○ | ○ |
| 6 | The department leads and senior management would support our teams to prescribe one unit at a time and use restrictive transfusion thresholds. | ○ | ○ | ○ | ○ | ○ |
| 7 | A restrictive RBC transfusion strategy is important for our patients. | ○ | ○ | ○ | ○ | ○ |
| 8 | Adopting a restrictive transfusion strategy would not come at the cost of improving other patient outcomes (e.g. slowing time to recovery or discharge). | ○ | ○ | ○ | ○ | ○ |
| 9 | It isn't my responsibility to ensure we transfuse one unit at a time and use restrictive transfusion thresholds. | ○ | ○ | ○ | ○ | ○ |
| 10 | I am not clear about what my role should be in the process to ensure we transfuse one unit at a time and use transfusion thresholds. | ○ | ○ | ○ | ○ | ○ |
| 11 | It will be bad for the patient if our team orders more than one unit at a time and uses liberal transfusion thresholds. | ○ | ○ | ○ | ○ | ○ |
| 12 | If our team orders more than one unit at a time and uses liberal transfusion thresholds, the negative consequences outweigh the good. | ○ | ○ | ○ | ○ | ○ |

*Source:* Choosing Wisely Canada; http://www.usingbloodwisely.ca/intervention.

## ANALYSING THE DATA

Once you have collected your data regarding the barriers to de-implementing low-value care, you now must analyse, group, and prioritise the barriers identified. The way in which you collect your data will guide your analysis process to identify barriers to de-implementing low-value care.

The qualitative analyses of interviews and focus group data can be done inductively, where you identify common themes across the interviews and observations through thematic analysis, or deductively using a framework approach. One benefit of using the TDF to guide the analysis approach is that it can help simplify the amount of data to work with by applying a deductive approach to the analysis (Atkins et al. 2017). When identifying what themes or domain are important to changing healthcare provider behaviour it is recommended you consider three factors: presence of conflicting beliefs, perceived strength of the beliefs impacting the behaviour, and frequency of the beliefs across interviews (Patey et al. 2012). However, frequency count of theme occurrence is not warranted in the case of focus group interviews as nonverbal agreement or disagreement with a fellow participant would not always be captured (Atkins et al. 2017). All three factors should be considered concurrently in establishing domain or theme importance.

Data collected via survey or questionnaire should be analysed using quantitative methods. A simple method of analysis could include calculating mean scores for the items of your survey such as shown in Box 8.5. More complex analysis may include regression analysis (Huijg et al. 2014). Scientific training or cooperation with methodologists or statisticians is recommended for the more complex analysis and interpretation of findings appropriately.

## NARROWING DOWN THE DRIVERS OR BARRIERS IDENTIFIED

It is unlikely that you will be able to address all the barriers to de-implementing low-value care identified by the healthcare providers, when developing your intervention. You will need to narrow the scope. There are several factors that may help guide your selection of barriers to which target:

1. What barriers are likely to have the greatest impact if removed or alleviated? Clinically, your participants in the data collection are the experts in the clinical practice behaviour, and if a barrier was repeatedly mentioned by them, it is likely an important one.

2. Can you address multiple barriers at once? Multiple barriers that can be targeted by one strategy may be easier to address than developing an intervention with multiple components targeting multiple barriers.

3. Are there barriers that may be easier to address than others? Barriers that are more amenable to change and likely require fewer resources may be easier to address than barriers that require copious resources.

These three factors are likely not the only things you need to consider, but it is a start. Team consensus can support priority setting. Chapter 9 will provide a more detailed discussion about how to select the de-implementation strategies or components to design your de-implementation intervention.

## KEY POINTS

- Specifying target behaviours and identifying the barriers for de-implementation is an important phase for designing a tailor-made intervention.
- We have provided some theory- and evidence-based tools to help you specify the behaviour that needs to change and identify the barriers that need to be targeted in a de-implementation intervention. We also present methods of data collection and analysis.
- Both in-depth qualitative explorations and observational studies should be used but will depend on resources and capacity. Interviews and direct observations are useful for the in-depth exploration of situations.

- For practical purposes, you will have to prioritise barriers you want to target in a de-implementation intervention. We have provided several factors to guide prioritisation.

## USEFUL RESOURCES

- The AACTT tool: https://static-content.springer.com/esm/art%3A10.1186%2Fs13012-019-0951-x/MediaObjects/13012_2019_951_MOESM1_ESM.pdf
- TDF series for interview guides: https://www.biomedcentral.com/collections/tdf
- Using Blood Wisely Survey: http://www.usingbloodwisely.ca/intervention

## REFERENCES

Atkins, L., Francis, J., Islam, R. et al. (2017). A guide to using the Theoretical Domains Framework of behaviour change to investigate implementation problems. *Implementation Science* 12: 77.

Bussières, A.E., Patey, A.M., Francis, J.J. et al. (2012). Identifying theory-based factors likely to influence compliance with diagnostic imaging guideline recommendations for spine disorders among chiropractors in North America: Qualitative study. *Implementation Science* 7:82. doi: 10.1186/1748-5908-7-8222938135

Cane, J., O'Connor, D., and Michie, S. (2012). Validation of the theoretical domains framework for use in behaviour change and implementation research. *Implementation Science* 7: 37.

Colquhoun, H., Grimshaw, J., and Wensing, M. (2013). Mapping KT interventions to barriers and facilitators. In: *Knowledge Translation in Health Care: Moving from Evidence to Practice* (ed. S.E. Straus, J. Tetroe, and I.D. Graham). Chichester: Wiley Blackwell.

Davis, R., Campbell, R., Hildon, Z. et al. (2014). Theories of behaviour and behaviour change across the social and behavioural sciences: a scoping review. *Health Psychology Review* 9: 323–344.

Dobson, G., Filteau, L., Fuda, G. et al. (2021). Guidelines to the practice of anesthesia – revised edition 2022 [Guide d'exercice de l'anesthésie de la SCA – Édition révisée 2022]. *Canadian Journal of Anaesthesia* 69: 1–38.

Eccles, M.P., Grimshaw, J.M., Johnston, M. et al. (2007). Applying psychological theories to evidence-based clinical practice: identifying factors predictive of managing upper respiratory tract infections without antibiotics. *Implementation Science* 2: 26.

Francis, J.J., Johnston, M., Robertson, C. et al. (2010). What is an adequate sample size? Operationalising data saturation for theory-based interview studies. *Psychology and Health* 25: 1229–1245.

French, S.D., Green, S., O'Connor, D. et al. (2012). Developing theory-informed behaviour change interventions to implement evidence into practice: a systematic approach using the theoretical domains framework. *Implementation Science* 7: 38.

Grimshaw, J.M., Eccles, M.P., Steen, N. et al. (2011). Applying psychological theories to evidence-based clinical practice: identifying factors predictive of lumbar spine x-ray for low back pain in UK primary care practice. *Implementation Science* 6: 55.

Grimshaw, J.M., Patey, A.M., Kirkham, K.R. et al. (2020). De-implementing wisely: developing the evidence base to reduce low-value care. *BMJ Quality and Safety* https://doi.org/10.1136/bmjqs-2019-010060.

Huijg, J.M., Gebhardt, W.A., Crone, M.R. et al. (2014). Discriminant content validity of a theoretical domains framework questionnaire for use in implementation research. *Implementation Science* 9: 1–16.

Islam, R., Tinmouth, A.T., Francis, J.J. et al. (2012). A cross-country comparison of intensive care physicians' beliefs about their transfusion behaviour: a qualitative study using the theoretical domains framework. *Implementation Science* 7: 93–93.

Lee, C., Jafari, M., Brownbridge, R. et al. (2020). The viral prescription pad-a mixed methods study to determine the need for and utility of an educational tool for antimicrobial stewardship in primary health care. *BMC Family Practice* 21: 1–12.

Michie, S., Richardson, M., Johnston, M. et al. (2013). The behavior change technique taxonomy (v1) of 93 hierarchically clustered techniques: building an international consensus for the reporting of behavior change interventions. *Annals of Behavioral Medicine* 46: 81–95.

Oeffinger, K.C., Fontham, E.T., Etzioni, R. et al. (2015). Breast cancer screening for women at average risk: 2015 guideline update from the American Cancer Society. *The Journal of the American Medical Association* 314: 1599–1614.

Patey, A.M., Islam, R., Francis, J.J. et al. (2012). Anesthesiologists' and surgeons' perceptions about routine pre-operative testing in low-risk patients: application of the Theoretical Domains Framework (TDF) to identify factors that influence physicians' decisions to order pre-operative tests. *Implementation Science* 7: 52.

Patey, A.M., Curran, J.A., Sprague, A.E. et al. (2017). Intermittent auscultation versus continuous fetal monitoring: exploring factors that influence birthing unit nurses' fetal surveillance practice using theoretical domains framework. *BMC Pregnancy and Childbirth* 17: 320.

Presseau, J., McCleary, N., Lorencatto, F. et al. (2019). Action, actor, context, target, time (AACTT): a framework for specifying behaviour. *Implementation Science* 14: 1–13.

Prothero, L., Lawrenson, J.G., Cartwright, M. et al. (2021). Barriers and enablers to diabetic eye screening attendance: an interview study with young adults with type 1 diabetes. *Diabetic Medicine* 39: e14751.

Sniehotta, F.F., Araújo-Soares, V., Brown, J. et al. (2017). Complex systems and individual-level approaches to population health: a false dichotomy? *The Lancet Public Health* 2: e396–e397.

Wang, V., Maciejewski, M.L., Helfrich, C.D. et al. (2018). Working smarter not harder: coupling implementation to de-implementation. *Healthcare* 6: 104–107.

# APPENDIX: SAMPLE INTERVIEW GUIDE FOR HEALTHCARE PROVIDERS USING THE TDF

*Please note that the text in Bold and Italics is for the interviewer only*

## Introduction Script

Thank you for agreeing to participate in this interview. The purpose of this interview is to understand the barriers and enablers you face when [BEHAVIOUR] and care for your patients.

Our discussion will be audio-recorded and transcribed, and the transcription will be cleared of any identifying information. The results will be published in such a way that your responses cannot be traced back to you. If you prefer not to answer a question, or would like to withdraw at any time, you are free to do so. Feel free to give examples if it helps you answer a question.

I am not a healthcare provider, nor am I here to make any clinical judgements. I just want to get a sense of your views and experiences. There are no right or wrong answers.

Is this ok with you? Circle: YES NO (Note: if no, do not proceed with interview)

Do you have any questions before we start?

---

NOTE THAT RECORDING WILL START NOW

## Background

I'd like to start with some basic questions:

1. What is your role/title?
2. What kind of setting do you work at (e.g. family health team, private clinic, and hospital)?
3. How long have you been working in your current position?
4. What percentage of your patients identify as [characteristic under investigation]?

For the rest of our conversation, I have some specific questions that focus on [BEHAVIOUR]. In answering these questions, I would like you to think about the following specific behaviour:

**Behaviour Under Investigation Using the AACTT**

Actor:

Action:

Target:

Time:

Context:

If at any point, you would like me to repeat this description of the behaviour, please let me know.

Some questions may seem repetitive, but please bear with me as they do try to get at slightly different things that may influence this behaviour.

If you are ready, we can start.

5. Could you walk me through the current process for [BEHAVIOUR]? (*PROMPT:* Can you describe the steps (that would be) involved from start to finish?

## Knowledge

*(WHAT DO THEY KNOW, AND HOW DOES THAT INFLUENCE WHAT THEY DO?)*

6. What is your understanding of [BEHAVIOUR]? What are your thoughts on it?
   - *PROMPT:* Are you familiar with all the steps involved?
7. Do you use/have any guidelines or policies for it?
   - If yes, which guidelines/policies, and what do they recommend?
   - If no, what do you use to guide your practice?

## Social/professional role and identity

*(HOW DOES WHO THEY ARE AS A HEALTHCARE PROVIDER INFLUENCE WHETHER THEY DO SOMETHING OR NOT?)*

8. What role do you play in the [BEHAVIOUR]?
9. Is there anything in your professional role that influences you to [BEHAVIOUR]?
   - *PROMPT*: professional training, guidelines, other technologies

10. Who else is involved to make sure that these procedures happen?

11. Would you see it as part of your job/responsibility to [BEHAVIOUR]?

12. Are there others who should be involved? Who should be involved, why, and how? Would you anticipate any problems arising?

## Skills

*(WHAT DO THEY KNOW ABOUT HOW THEY SHOULD BE DOING SOMETHING AND HOW DOES THAT INFLUENCE WHETHER THEY DO IT OR NOT?)*

13. What expertise does someone in your role need to [BEHAVIOUR]?

14. Do you think that you have the necessary expertise to [BEHAVIOUR]? If not, what could help?

15. Is there any additional training you think you would need to [BEHAVIOUR]? Or that you think other people you work with would benefit from? What would that be?

## Beliefs about capabilities

*(DO THEY THINK THAT THEY CAN DO WHAT THEY SHOULD DO AND HOW DOES THAT INFLUENCE WHETHER THEY DO IT OR NOT?)*

16. How easy or difficult is it for you to [BEHAVIOUR]? What would make it easier?
    - *PROMPT*: What makes it easy? Why?
    - *PROMPT*: What makes it difficult? Why?

17. How confident do you feel in your ability to [BEHAVIOUR]? What makes you feel less confident/what would make you feel more confident?

18. How much personal control do you think you have over your ability to [BEHAVIOUR]? What things would influence your use that are beyond your control? What would increase your control?

## Optimism

*(HOW DOES WHETHER THEY ARE OPTIMISTIC/ PESSIMISTIC INFLUENCE WHAT THEY DO?)*

19. How optimistic are you that [BEHAVIOUR] will help you/ your patients/overall? Why?
    - *PROMPT*: level of optimism high/low?

## Beliefs about consequences

*(WHAT ARE THE GOOD AND BAD THINGS THAT CAN HAPPEN FROM WHAT THEY DO AND HOW DOES THAT INFLUENCE WHETHER THEY'LL DO IT IN THE FUTURE?)*

20. What do you think are be the benefits or positive impacts of [BEHAVIOUR]?
    - *PROMPT*: For yourself, your patients, your colleagues, your setting, other people in the community?
    - *PROMPT*: Impact on workload?
21. Are there any harms or negative impacts that you think may occur from [BEHAVIOUR]?
    - *PROMPT*: For yourself, your patients, your colleagues, your setting, other people in the community?
    - *PROMPT*: Impact on workload? Costs?
22. Do the potential benefits of [BEHAVIOUR] outweigh the potential harms? If not, what could help achieve this?

## Reinforcement

*(HOW HAVE THEIR EXPERIENCES (GOOD AND BAD) OF DOING IT IN THE PAST INFLUENCE WHETHER OR NOT THEY DO IT?)*

23. How have previous experiences of doing [BEHAVIOUR] impact you plan to do [BEHAVIOUR] in the future?
    - *PROMPT*: Bad experience = not going to [BEHAVIOUR], positive experience = likely to do it again
24. Are there any incentives or rewarding experiences that encourages/would encourage you to [BEHAVIOUR]?
25. Are there any/Can you foresee any sanctions that may be associated with [BEHAVIOUR]?

## Intention

*(HOW DOES HOW INCLINED THEY ARE TO DO SOMETHING INFLUENCE WHETHER THEY WILL DO IT?)*

26. To what extent do you want/intend to [BEHAVIOUR]?
    - *PROMPT*: In what situations may you find yourself more motivated? Why?
    - *PROMPT*: In what situations may you find yourself less motivated? Why?

## Goals

*(HOW IMPORTANT IS WHAT THEY DO AND DOES THAT INFLUENCE WHETHER OR NOT THEY DO IT? WHAT STANDARDS ARE THEY TRYING TO REACH, HOW DOES THAT INFLUENCE WHETHER OR NOT THEY DO IT?)*

27. How important is it for you to [BEHAVIOUR]?

28. Is [BEHAVIOUR] something that you feel you would want or need to do? What would drive that?

29. Thinking about all your other tasks in the healthcare setting, how much of a priority is it for you to [BEHAVIOUR] compared to other priorities that you may have?

   - *PROMPT*: Why is/is not it a priority?

### Memory, attention, and decision processes

*(HOW DOES THEIR FORGETFULNESS OR REMEMBERING TO DO IT INFLUENCE WHETHER OR NOT THEY DO IT?*

*HOW DOES THEIR ABILITY TO FOCUS ON THE BEHAVIOUR INFLUENCE WHETHER OR NOT THEY DO IT? HOW DO THE DECISIONS THEY MAKE ABOUT THE BEHAVIOUR INFLUENCE WHETHER THEY DO IT OR NOT?)*

30. Is [BEHAVIOUR] an automatic or routine part of your work, or is it be something you need to stop and take time to think about?

31. In what situations do/would you decide to [BEHAVIOUR]? Why?

32. In what situations might you decide not to [BEHAVIOUR]? Why? What would you do instead?

### Environmental context and resources

*(WHAT ARE THE THINGS IN THEIR ENVIRONMENT THAT INFLUENCE WHAT THEY DO AND HOW DO THEY INFLUENCE? NOT JUST PHYSICAL STUFF, BUT ACCESS TO OTHER PROFESSIONALS)*

33. What aspects of your setting influence you in [BEHAVIOUR]?

    Are there competing tasks/demands or time constraints that interferes with [BEHAVIOUR]? What are they? What could help overcome them?

34. Are there any additional resources you would need to [BEHAVIOUR]?

    - **PROMPT**: To what extent are additional resources needed available?

## Social Influences

*(WHAT DO OTHERS THINK OF WHAT THEY DO? WHO ARE THEY AND HOW DOES THAT INFLUENCE WHAT THEY DO?)*

35. Who influences your likelihood of [BEHAVIOUR], and how?

    - **PROMPT**: Colleagues; residents/trainees; your patients; managers; others?

36. How might the views or opinions of others affect you to [BEHAVIOUR]?

37. Do your colleagues agree with what you do in your practice with respect [BEHAVIOUR]? Do they have similar procedures or not?

## Emotion

*(HOW DO THEY FEEL ABOUT WHAT THEY DO AND DO THOSE FEELINGS INFLUENCE WHAT THEY DO?)*

38. Do you have any worries or concerns about [BEHAVIOUR]?

39. How do you feel about [BEHAVIOUR] (when you think of [BEHAVIOUR], what sorts of emotions come to mind)?

    - **PROMPT**: anxiety, stress, positive emotion?

## Behavioural regulation

*(WHAT DO THEY THINK WOULD HELP/WHAT STRATEGIES HAVE HELPED THEM DO WHAT YOU SHOULD DO? WHAT STRATEGIES ARE ALREADY IN PLACE TO HELP THEM DO WHAT THEY SHOULD DO?)*

40. What strategies, supports, or ways of working do you have in place that help you in [BEHAVIOUR]?
41. If you wanted to implement changes in your own practice setting to encourage [BEHAVIOUR], what would be some ways to do this?

Those are all the questions I have for you. I appreciate the time and insight that you have given me today. Is there anything else related to this topic you would like to talk about that we have not covered? Thank you!

# CHAPTER 9

# Selecting De-Implementation Strategies and Designing Interventions: Phase 2b

Justin Presseau[1,2,3], Nicola McCleary[1,2,3,4], Andrea M. Patey[1,2,3], Sheena McHugh[5], and Fabiana Lorencatto[6]

[1] Clinical Epidemiology Program, Ottawa Hospital Research Institute, Ottawa, Ontario, Canada
[2] School of Epidemiology and Public Health, University of Ottawa, Ottawa, Ontario, Canada
[3] Centre for Implementation Research, Ottawa Hospital Research Institute, Ottawa, Ontario, Canada
[4] Eastern Ontario Regional Laboratory Association, Ottawa, Ontario, Canada
[5] School of Public Health, University College Cork, Western Gateway Building, Cork, Ireland
[6] Centre for Behaviour Change, University College London, London, UK

*How to Reduce Overuse in Healthcare: A Practical Guide*, First Edition.
Edited by Tijn Kool, Andrea M. Patey, Simone van Dulmen, and Jeremy M. Grimshaw.
© 2024 John Wiley & Sons Ltd. Published 2024 by John Wiley & Sons Ltd.

## WHAT DO YOU NEED TO DO BEFORE SELECTING DE-IMPLEMENTATION STRATEGIES?

As outlined in earlier chapters, developing de-implementation interventions is greatly aided by a thorough understanding of the determinants of the prioritised low-value care and of barriers and enablers to its de-implementation. Further, linking the evidence of barriers and enablers to an existing framework, such as the ones outlined in Chapter 8, provides you with an advantage by helping you to identify which de-implementation strategies are – or are not – best fit to address those issues. Much as we may wish it to be so, there are rarely 'magic bullets' or one-size-fits-all strategies that work for all low-value practices in all settings. Frameworks that match strategies to different types of barriers and enablers provide an evidence-based foundation to help get you started. That is not to say that starting from scratch does not have its merits. But doing so risks a potentially time-consuming and expensive exercise of trial and error. Indeed, using frameworks and theories is a way to build on what is already known, so that you can focus your expertise and resources as you develop and optimise the de-implementation intervention for your context.

This chapter is designed to provide practical advice, offering 10 general principles to consider as you select strategies to inform the design of your de-implementation interventions. We provide key accessible tools for each principle.

## TEN GENERAL PRINCIPLES TO CONSIDER AS YOU DEVELOP A DE-IMPLEMENTATION INTERVENTION

### 1. There Are No Magic Bullets: Design Your De-Implementation Intervention to Address Specific Barriers and Enablers

If there was a universally effective de-implementation strategy, you would not be reading this book. While there is evidence for the effectiveness of many broadly-defined strategies (e.g. audit and feedback, educational outreach, and continuing professional development), the state of the evidence for many of these broad strategies has moved beyond 'does this work' and more to 'when does this work, for whom, under what circumstances' (Ivers et al. 2014). The implication then is that by jumping to de-implementation strategies before understanding the contextual and reinforcing factors that maintain existing low-value care, you risk developing a solution not matched to the problem, as described in Chapter 8. This first principle is, thus, a redoubled call for making sure that the strategies you select to de-implement the low-value care of interest are designed to address the known barriers and drivers of the care you are seeking to change.

## 2. De-Implementation Interventions Are Often Also Implementation Interventions when Substituting One Practice with Another

Healthcare professionals have been trained and developed competencies and expertise to intervene to help, as will be discussed in Chapter 12. In some ways, the very idea of reducing or stopping an existing practice, especially one driven by habits and routines, runs counter to this training and expertise. If you are reading this book, you are likely of the view that reducing or stopping low-value care is part and parcel of health professionals' commitment to providing the best possible up-to-date care to their patients. But that does not necessarily make it any easier for someone whose career and everyday experience is more typically about *doing something*, not about the *absence of doing something*. Thus, a unique feature of de-implementation interventions, compared to implementation interventions to introduce a new practice or improve an existing practice, is the opportunity to promote alternative practices as a substitute for the low-value care that you seek to reduce. For instance, in Chapter 3, we identified alternatives to acid-reducing medication for babies experiencing persistent crying. Indeed, the strategy of 'Behavioural substitution' is very frequently used in de-implementation interventions (Patey et al. 2021). It is not a given that merely suggesting an alternative will be sufficient to reduce the momentum of well-ingrained practices, so it is important to *also* consider how to promote the implementation of that new, alternative practice. You should then consider treating the alternative practice behaviour as a second target for your intervention, where you need to develop an implementation intervention to promote the use of that alternative behaviour. That second target would also benefit from a clearer understanding of any barriers and enablers to its use.

## 3. Routinised, Habitually Performed Care May Be Operating Semi-Automatically

Some low-value care may be well-entrenched and part of routine practice, thus not relying as much on a need to weigh every decision, as we explained in Chapters 2 and 3. An example is routine preoperative test ordering for day surgery or daily lab tests for patients in hospital (Kirkham et al. 2015). If part of your strategy is to replace a routinised low-value care with a new alternative that is not embedded or routinised yet as explained above in principle 2, you might need two different strategies: one to disrupt the routinised behaviour using strategies that address the automaticity of that existing practice, and another to encourage the uptake of its alternative which likely is not yet operating in the same semi-automatic way. If you identify factors that drive current low-value care that are largely routinely or automatically performed, make sure you consider strategies that are specifically designed to disrupt automatic/semi-automatic behaviours (Potthoff et al. 2022). These are different from educational and guideline-based strategies. For instance, Learning Theory (Skinner 1963) proposes that strategies providing a reward contingent on performance of an action are a powerful source of producing more automatic decisions and actions. Seeking and reducing existing behaviour-reward contingencies may help to reduce the routine action. Note that rewards need not be financial; e.g. social rewards from leadership and colleagues can also serve as contingent rewards. Social cues in the work setting can also serve to keep an automatic behaviour going, for example, if someone regularly prompts another health professional to engage in the low-value care; part of the solution in that instance involves identifying what those social prompts and cues are and reducing their use. Similarly, physical and/or electronic prompts and cues may contribute to prompting the low-value care you seek to reduce and could also be altered. Examples are reminders or flags in an electronic medical record or the composition of an ordering form or the setup of the rooms in which the low-value care is delivered. Audit and feedback can also serve as part of an automaticity-disruptive strategy in some cases, especially where the recipient is unaware of the degree to which they are performing the low-value care. There are many other approaches, but the general principle here is that if the low-value care you are seeking to reduce involves performance that is operating semi-automatically, be sure to consider strategies that are specific to addressing that automaticity.

## 4. Follow the Evidence Wherever Possible when Designing Your De-Implementation Intervention

As you develop your de-implementation intervention, consider what is already known about the effectiveness of the strategies that you are considering. Doing so has the advantage of maximising the evidenced-informed selection of strategies and ensuring that you are not spending your time 'reinventing the wheel' instead of focusing on how to optimise your intervention. One key resource is the Cochrane Effective Practice and Organisation of Care (EPOC) Group (see sources at the end of the chapter) that supports dozens of systematic reviews of a range of implementation strategies, some of which have been evaluated dozens if not hundreds of times across a range of healthcare settings and clinical topics using (cluster) randomised designs (see Table 9.1). While there may not be a systematic review for every de-implementation strategy that you are considering, it is worth assessing those that do have rigorous evidence supporting them as part of your strategy selection process (Potthoff et al. 2018).

**TABLE 9.1**   Effectiveness of a selection of trialled implementation strategies synthesised in Cochrane EPOC reviews.

| Implementation strategy synthesised in Cochrane review | Total number of randomised trials | Median improvement in clinical practice[a] (%) |
| --- | --- | --- |
| Printed educational materials (Giguère et al. 2020) | 32 | 4 (IQR 1–9) |
| Computerised clinical decision support systems (Kwan et al. 2020)[b] | 122 | 5.8 (95 CI 4.0–7.6) |
| Manually generated paper-based reminders (Pantoja et al. 2019) | 59 | 8.5 (IQR 2.5–20.6) |
| Computer-generated paper-based reminders (Arditi et al. 2017) | 30 | 6.8 (IQR 3.8–17.5) |
| Audit and feedback (Ivers et al. 2012) | 140 | 4.3 (IQR 0.5–16) |
| Continuing education meetings and workshops (Forsetlund et al. 2021) | 215 | 4 (IQR 0.3–13) |
| Local opinion leaders (Flodgren et al. 2019) | 18 | 10.8 (IQR 3.5–14.6) |
| Educational outreach visits (O'Brien et al. 2007) | 69 | 5.6 (IQR 3–9) |

[a] Based on primary dichotomous analysis reported
[b] Update of a previous Cochrane review

## 5. Avoid the Tower of Babel: Leverage Existing Lists of Change Strategies and Use Them to Help Match Specific Strategies to Identified Barriers/Enablers

Given the range of possible strategies available, it is important to guard against using the same term to describe different strategies or different terms to describe the same strategy. That is not to dissuade you from coining a new term for your strategy, but if you do, make sure that there is not an existing strategy known by a different term being used already. Thankfully, there are already lists of strategies that have been collated and agreed, with definitions and examples of how each strategy is used. Below you can find three complementary lists to consider as part of your strategy selection toolkit. They are also highlighted at the end of the chapter as potential sources of information including where to find them.

a. *Cochrane EPOC Taxonomy*: underpins the evidence in Cochrane EPOC reviews and includes strategies across four key domains of health system interventions: delivery arrangements, financial arrangements, governance arrangements, and implementation strategies (Effective Practice and Organization of Care 2015). The taxonomy describes a range of specific strategies within each of those four domains and provides definitions for each. Perhaps uniquely, relative to other similar lists, there are Cochrane EPOC reviews of the effectiveness of many of the strategies outlined (see Table 9.1 for examples), thus providing you with the ability to leverage the evidence in support (or not) of particular strategies as part of your decisions to select a given de-implementation strategy.

b. *Expert Recommendations for Implementing Change (ERIC)*: The ERIC taxonomy compiles 73 implementation strategies into nine groups, providing labels and definitions for each (Powell et al. 2015; Waltz et al. 2015).

c. *Behaviour Change Techniques Taxonomy and Behaviour Change Wheel (BCW)*: The BCW is a framework that at its core describes the capability, opportunity, and motivation-related barriers and enablers from the Theoretical Domains Framework (see Chapter 8). It links them to nine types of strategies, which can be supported by seven policy levers. The BCW neatly links the barriers to strategies, through to policy supports needed to enact the strategies. However, as these nine strategies are broadly specified, it can help to 'dig deeper' into the range of more elemental techniques underpinned by each of the nine strategies. The complementary Behaviour Change Techniques Taxonomy does just that: it is a list of 93 ways of changing behaviour that can be applied across settings including de-implementation (Patey et al. 2021) and implementation (Konnyu et al. 2020) interventions. It is also possible to use the EPOC taxonomy or ERIC taxonomy as the higher-level description of strategies and the Behaviour Change Techniques Taxonomy as a content-specific strategy descriptor (Konnyu et al. 2020; McHugh et al. 2022).

Given the range of strategies available, a key challenge is how to choose from amongst these options. This is where the value of identifying barriers and enablers, as suggested from Chapter 8, shines. For the ERIC, BCT, and BCW lists, there are tools available that directly link specific strategies to specific barriers and enablers frameworks to help in deciding which strategies are fit for addressing which barriers, and which are not. For example, each barrier and enabler categorised in the Theoretical Domains Framework (Atkins et al. 2017) is linked to specific intervention strategies and policy enablers in the BCW (Michie et al. 2011). Tools such as the 'Theory and Techniques Tool' provide another link between barriers and enablers from the Theoretical Domains Framework to the Behaviour Change Techniques best suited to address them (Centre for Behaviour Change 2019). Similarly, the Consolidated Framework for Implementation Research (CFIR), another commonly used framework for identifying barriers and enablers, includes a tool to match CFIR-identified barriers to specific ERIC taxonomy strategies best suited to address those barriers (Waltz et al. 2019). It is important to note that these tools that link barriers to fit-for-purpose strategies serve to more quickly narrow the vast possible options of strategies that you could choose down to those that might be especially well suited to address barriers and enablers to reducing low-value care in your setting.

## 6. Avoid Conflating Intervention Content with Its Method of Delivery

When developing a de-implementation intervention, there are decisions to be made about the content but also how that content will be delivered: the mode of delivery. Consider a pharmaceutical analogy: the active ingredients of a pharmaceutical therapy (i.e., the drug) designed to provide pain relief is not the same as the range of ways in which that active content can be delivered to achieve its effect (e.g., by tablet, injection, or suppository). Similarly, a de-implementation intervention can be delivered in many ways, e.g. in-person or virtual meeting, outreach visit to a practice, online or in person, self-directed or facilitated, using videos or PowerPoint, paper or electronic, or through an app. Pinning down the ways in which your de-implementation intervention will be delivered is important, but it is critical to not assume that the way that you deliver your de-implementation intervention is the intervention strategy. Instead, think about intervention strategy content, that is, *what* you will do as part of the intervention, separately from *how* that content will be delivered (Hoffmann et al. 2014). Often, the temptation is to gravitate towards describing an intervention strategy by how it is delivered ('develop an app', 'provide education', or 'develop and disseminate a guideline'). We encourage you to make the distinction between 'what to deliver' and 'how to deliver it'. Making that distinction helps to select which sets of de-implementation strategies are best suited to address the barriers to change (see principles 4 and 5 above for ideas of where to look for describing the 'what' of your strategy). Then, select the mode(s) of delivery that ensures that the content of your intervention reaches your intended audience, is feasibly delivered within yours and your recipients' available resources, and is acceptable. The distinction between content and mode of delivery is increasingly recognised in tools such as guidance for how best to report intervention descriptions so that others can repeat it (Hoffmann et al. 2014; Pinnock et al. 2017).

## 7. Decide on Tailoring and Adaptation

At a high level, the entire process of matching barriers and enablers to implementation strategies is itself a form of tailoring an intervention, that is, of matching solutions to known reasons for low-value care (Baker et al. 2015; Powell et al. 2017). However, here, we focus specifically on tailoring and adapting your delivery and intervention content to account for variations in patient mix, clinicians, or organisation(s) in which your intervention is to be delivered. It may be important for some strategies of your de-implementation intervention to be consistently delivered to everyone in a similar way, whilst other strategies in your intervention may benefit from being tailored to the individual clinicians, settings, and/or organisations receiving the intervention. If you decide that one or more strategies would benefit from being tailored at this level, the key is clearly specifying what will be tailored and how it will work before the intervention is delivered. Once the intervention is being delivered, changes may crop up – e.g., the person delivering the intervention may have to change, or a feedback report may need to be delivered more or less frequently in some settings once you get going. Such changes can happen and are typically seen as 'adaptations' where the need to pivot only becomes apparent once you start delivering the intervention, rather than tailored parts of the intervention which are the pre-planned ways in which you want your intervention and its strategies to be delivered differently to its recipients depending on prespecified criteria (Hoffmann et al. 2014).

## 8. Co-Development, User-Centred Design to Enhance Feasibility, Acceptability, and Implementability

Developing de-implementation interventions cannot be (solely) a desk-based exercise. Iteration and engaging with multidisciplinary expertise including clinical, implementation science, quality improvement, organisational, and lived experience expertise (including patients as discussed in Chapter 5), can ensure the feasibility, acceptability, and implementability of your intervention (Klaic et al. 2022). Make sure to build in time to iterate the intervention development, which can be aided by using a logic model (see principle 10). Where possible, and especially if your de implementation intervention involves materials such as an app to download and navigate, a dashboard to consult, a feedback report to consider or an email to open, it can be useful to watch a diverse group of health providers (who are ideally not part of your team per se) and patients interact with and give their perspectives on prototypes of materials. Ultimately, these processes can help to inform strategy selection and piloting your de-implementation with a diversity of recipients. This step can help to iron out any assumptions that you have made, ultimately helping you to sleep better at night ahead of launching the actual intervention in the knowledge that you have assessed whether your intervention can be feasibly delivered, is acceptable to those engaging with it, and that it can be delivered as designed.

## 9. Prioritise Equity

De-implementation interventions are inherently designed to improve upon current care, removing care that is of less value, and, in some instances, replacing that care with better evidenced, higher value care. We sincerely doubt anyone designing de-implementation interventions wilfully ignores equity. But without putting effort into ensuring equity, there is a risk that your well-intentioned de-implementation intervention ultimately only de-implements low-value care for a subgroup whose circumstances enable them to benefit, thereby leaving others to continue to deliver and/or receive low-value care (Brownson et al. 2021). The result is a risk for de-implementation intervention-generated inequities. Carefully consider where your de-implementation intervention will be evaluated and/or delivered. Ensure wherever possible that the sites at which your intervention is delivered at least include those providing care to a diversity of patients. Consider equity in as many steps as possible of your de-implementation intervention design and deployment.

This begins in the formation of your intervention design team to help surface and mitigate any potential unidentified consequences that might lead to differential effects of your de-implementation intervention (see principle 8). Your design team should ideally include representation from a diversity of patients whose care would be affected by your intervention, as described in Chapter 5. Your design team should ideally also include representation from clinicians practicing in diverse settings (e.g. including rural and/or non-academic healthcare centres, serving a diversity of populations) and clinicians spanning a range of intersecting personal characteristics. Prioritising equity also involves considering how and by whom your de-implementation intervention will be delivered and to whom: healthcare settings are a microcosm of society; teams of healthcare providers involve people across sexes and genders, races and ethnicities, sexual orientations, ages, and degrees of professional and social capital that can produce power dynamics and hierarchies. These lived realities of health providers may contribute to barriers and enablers to de-implementing, or indeed for the intended healthcare professional recipients of your de-implementation intervention being able to engage in your intervention at all. Consider also using tools that acknowledge these factors as part of the frameworks highlighted in this and other chapters. This can be further aided by piloting your developed de-implementation intervention with a diversity of health providers to assess the feasibility, acceptability (Sekhon et al. 2017), and implementability of your intervention (Klaic et al. 2022). And you can use existing tools for measuring each of those (Kerkhoff et al. 2022; Presseau et al. 2022; Sibley et al. 2022).

## 10. Describe How the Strategy Works by Developing a De-Implementation Logic Model of Change

Given the number of possible moving parts in a de-implementation intervention, it can be helpful to surface the assumptions of how the intervention is expected to impact on the barriers and enablers to reducing low-value care. Developing a logic model, sometimes known as a program theory, can help to make explicit what is otherwise implicit by using a visual figure. This is helpful for ensuring that all stakeholders are on the same page about what the intervention will involve and how it is anticipated to work. Importantly, it can help others who may want to replicate, scale, and/or spread your intervention to have a clearer sense of how your de-implementation works. Davidoff et al. (2015) and Smith et al. (2020) do a nice job of exemplifying the range of ways that logic models can be developed and displayed. Logic models need not be complex: aim to visually describe (e.g. with boxes and arrows) which intervention strategies are included (using the taxonomies described above) to address which barriers and enablers (informed by frameworks, as described in Chapter 8) for which recipients of the intervention to achieve which changes in the behaviours implicated in the low-value care that you seek to reduce. The additional upshot of a logic model is that it provides a basis to keep track of the components of your interventions while you iterate it during development.

## KEY POINTS

- There are no de-implementation strategies that work all the time, but there are a wide range of strategies that you can choose from depending on barriers, feasibility, acceptability, and implementability considerations in your context.
- Draw from existing lists of (de)implementation strategies when selecting and operationalising instead of coining new terms.
- If your de-implementation intervention involves substituting one action for another, the substituted action should be the focus of a complementary implementation intervention.
- Explicitly describing your development process and defining your logic model will help you more fully understand

what works/does not work and why, to enable continual evidence accumulation on the best ways to de-implement low-value care for your own and other teams.

## SOURCES

- Template for intervention description and replication (TIDieR) (see Table 1): https://www.bmj.com/content/348/bmj.g1687
- Expert Recommendations for Implementing Change (ERIC) implementation strategy list (see Table 3): https://implementationscience.biomedcentral.com/articles/10.1186/s13012-015-0209-1
- Cochrane Effective Practice and Organisation of Care (EPOC) taxonomy of health systems interventions: https://epoc.cochrane.org/epoc-taxonomy
- Behaviour Change Wheel (see Tables for list of interventions and policies, and their links to framework-informed barriers/enablers of behaviour): https://implementationscience.biomedcentral.com/articles/10.1186/1748-5908-6-42
- Tool for mapping behaviour change techniques to determinants: https://theoryandtechniquetool.humanbehaviourchange.org
- Tool for developing de-implementation strategy logic model (see Fig 1 and 2 for examples): https://implementationscience.biomedcentral.com/articles/10.1186/s13012-020-01041-8

## REFERENCES

Arditi, C., Rège-Walther, M., Durieux, P. et al. (2017). Computer-generated reminders delivered on paper to healthcare professionals: effects on professional practice and healthcare outcomes. *Cochrane Database of Systematic Reviews* 7: (Art. No: CD001175).

Atkins, L., Francis, J., Islam, R. et al. (2017). A guide to using the theoretical domains framework of behaviour change to investigate implementation problems. *Implementation Science* 12: 77.

Baker, R., Camosso-Stefinovic, J., Gillies, C. et al. (2015). Tailored interventions to address determinants of practice. *Cochrane Database of Systematic Reviews* (Art. No: CD005470).

Brownson, R.C., Kumanyika, S.K., Kreuter, M.W. et al. (2021). Implementation science should give higher priority to health equity. *Implementation Science* 16: 28.

Centre for Behaviour Change. (2019). Theory and Techniques Tool. Theory and Techniques Tool. https://theoryandtechniquetool.humanbehaviourchange.org (accessed 15 April 2019).

Davidoff, F., Dixon-Woods, M., Leviton, L. et al. (2015). Demystifying theory and its use in improvement. *BMJ Quality & Safety* 24: 228–238.

Effective Practice and Organization of Care. (2015). EPOC Taxonomy. Norwegian Knowledge Centre for the Health Services. https://epoc.cochrane.org/epoc-taxonomy (accessed 15 May 2016).

Flodgren, G., O'Brien, M.A., Parmelli, E. et al. (2019). Local opinion leaders: effects on professional practice and healthcare outcomes. *Cochrane Database of Systematic Reviews* (Art. No: CD000125).

Forsetlund, L., O'Brien, M.A., Forsen, L. et al. (2021). Continuing education meetings and workshops: effects on professional practice and healthcare outcomes. *Cochrane Database of Systematic Reviews* (Art. No: CD003030).

Giguère, A., Zomahoun, H.T.V., Carmichael, P.-H. et al. (2020). Printed educational materials: effects on professional practice and healthcare outcomes. *Cochrane Database of Systematic Reviews* (Art. No: CD004398).

Hoffmann, T.C., Glasziou, P.P., Boutron, I. et al. (2014). Better reporting of interventions: template for intervention description and replication (TIDieR) checklist and guide. *British Medical Journal* 348: g1687.

Ivers, N., Jamtvedt, G., Flottorp, S. et al. (2012). Audit and feedback: effects on professional practice and healthcare outcomes. *Cochrane Database of Systematic Reviews* 6.

Ivers, N.M., Sales, A., Colquhoun, H. et al. (2014). No more 'business as usual' with audit and feedback interventions: towards an agenda for a reinvigorated intervention. *Implementation Science* 9: 14.

Kerkhoff, A.D., Farrand, E., Marquez, C. et al. (2022). Addressing health disparities through implementation science – a need to integrate an equity lens from the outset. *Implementation Science* 17: 13.

Kirkham, K.R., Wijeysundera, D.N., Pendrith, C. et al. (2015). Preoperative testing before low-risk surgical procedures. *Canadian Medical Association Journal* 187: E349–E358.

Klaic, M., Kapp, S., Hudson, P. et al. (2022). Implementability of healthcare interventions: an overview of reviews and development of a conceptual framework. *Implementation Science* 17: 10.

Konnyu, K.J., McCleary, N., Presseau, J. et al. (2020). Behavior change techniques in continuing professional development. *Journal of Continuing Education in the Health Professions* 40: 268–273.

Kwan, J.L., Lo, L., Ferguson, J. et al. (2020). Computerised clinical decision support systems and absolute improvements in care: meta-analysis of controlled clinical trials. *British Medical Journal* 370: m3216.

McHugh, S., Presseau, J., Luecking, C.T. et al. (2022). Examining the complementarity between the ERIC compilation of implementation strategies and the behaviour change technique taxonomy: a qualitative analysis. *Implementation Science* 17: 56.

Michie, S., van Stralen, M.M., and West, R. (2011). The behaviour change wheel: a new method for characterising and designing behaviour change interventions. *Implementation Science* 6: 42.

O'Brien, M.A., Rogers, S., Jamtvedt, G. et al. (2007). *Educational Outreach Visits: Effects on Professional Practice and Health Care Outcomes*. The Cochrane Library.

Pantoja, T., Grimshaw, J.M., Colomer, N. et al. (2019). Manually-generated reminders delivered on paper: effects on professional practice and patient outcomes. *Cochrane Database of Systematic Reviews* (Art. No: CD001174).

Patey, A.M., Grimshaw, J.M., and Francis, J.J. (2021). Changing behaviour, 'more or less': do implementation and de-implementation interventions include different behaviour change techniques? *Implementation Science* 16: 20.

Pinnock, H., Barwick, M., Carpenter, C.R. et al. (2017). Standards for reporting implementation studies (StaRI) statement. *British Medical Journal* 356: i6795.

Potthoff, S., McCleary, N., Sniehotta, F.F. et al. (2018). Creating and breaking habit in healthcare professional behaviours to improve healthcare and health. In: *The Psychology of Habit: Theory, Mechanisms, Change, and Contexts* (ed. B. Verplanken). Cham: Springer.

Potthoff, S., Kwasnicka, D., Avery, L. et al. (2022). Changing healthcare professionals' non-reflective processes to improve the quality of care. *Social Science & Medicine* 298: 114840.

Powell, B.J., Waltz, T.J., Chinman, M.J. et al. (2015). A refined compilation of implementation strategies: results from the expert recommendations for implementing change (ERIC) project. *Implementation Science* 10: 21.

Powell, B.J., Beidas, R.S., Lewis, C.C. et al. (2017). Methods to improve the selection and tailoring of implementation strategies. *The Journal of Behavioral Health Services & Research* 44: 177–194.

Presseau, J., Kasperavicius, D., Rodrigues, I.B. et al. (2022). Selecting implementation models, theories, and frameworks in which to integrate intersectional approaches. *BMC Medical Research Methodology* 22: 212.

Sekhon, M., Cartwright, M., and Francis, J.J. (2017). Acceptability of healthcare interventions: an overview of reviews and development of a theoretical framework. *BMC Health Services Research* 17: 88.

Sibley, K.M., Kasperavicius, D., Rodrigues, I.B. et al. (2022). Development and usability testing of tools to facilitate incorporating intersectionality in knowledge translation. *BMC Health Services Research* 22: 830.

Skinner, B.F. (1963). Operant Behavior. *American Psychologist* 18: 503.

Smith, J.D., Li, D.H., and Rafferty, M.R. (2020). The implementation research logic model: a method for planning, executing, reporting, and synthesizing implementation projects. *Implementation Science* 15: 84.

Waltz, T.J., Powell, B.J., Matthieu, M.M. et al. (2015). Use of concept mapping to characterize relationships among implementation strategies and assess their feasibility and importance: results from the Expert Recommendations for Implementing Change (ERIC) study. *Implementation Science* 10: 109.

Waltz, T.J., Powell, B.J., Fernández, M.E. et al. (2019). Choosing implementation strategies to address contextual barriers: diversity in recommendations and future directions. *Implementation Science* 14: 42.

# CHAPTER 10

# Evaluating De-Implementation Interventions: Phase 3

Beatriz Goulao[1], Eva W. Verkerk[2], Kednapa Thavorn[3,4,5], Justin Presseau[3,4,5], and Monica Taljaard[3,4,5]

[1] Health Services Research Unit, University of Aberdeen, Aberdeen, Scotland
[2] Department of IQ Healthcare, Radboud University Medical Center, Radboud Institute for Health Sciences, Nijmegen, The Netherlands
[3] Centre for Implementation Research, Ottawa Hospital Research Institute, Ottawa, Ontario, Canada
[4] School of Epidemiology and Public Health, University of Ottawa, Ottawa, Ontario, Canada
[5] Clinical Epidemiology Program, Ottawa Hospital Research Institute, Ottawa, Ontario, Canada

*How to Reduce Overuse in Healthcare: A Practical Guide*, First Edition.
Edited by Tijn Kool, Andrea M. Patey, Simone van Dulmen, and Jeremy M. Grimshaw.
© 2024 John Wiley & Sons Ltd. Published 2024 by John Wiley & Sons Ltd.

## WHY SHOULD WE EVALUATE?

De-implementation interventions require time and resources. For this reason, it is crucial to evaluate whether your intervention reduced low-value care and to monitor for unintended consequences (see Chapter 7). We also need to build the scientific basis for de-implementation (Grimshaw et al. 2020; Born et al. 2018).

The evaluation of de-implementation interventions can have two main purposes:

1. *programme evaluation and monitoring* to assess whether the intervention had its intended effects in your specific context contributing to local (organisational) knowledge;
2. *research evaluation* to produce generalisable knowledge about the effects of an intervention that contributes to scientific knowledge and can be used to spread interventions to different contexts. Research evaluation allows others to adopt potentially effective strategies.

Different evaluation purposes may need different evaluation methods. When evaluating an intervention, you may also consider what can be improved in the intervention, whether it worked better under certain conditions and whether the intervention was cost-effective. A well-performed evaluation could reassure and convince your team members and other stakeholders of the importance of further reducing the low-value care practice.

## OUTCOMES

A key aspect of evaluation is to define what aspects of clinical care the intervention aims to change, the outcomes of the intervention, and how they will be measured by outcome measures (for further discussion, see Chapter 7). Perhaps the most common outcome to measure is the reduction of low-value care such as the reduction in unnecessary medications prescribed by general practitioners (GPs). Other, indirect benefits from reducing the low-value care for the patient, healthcare professional, or the healthcare system could also be measured. These include clinical benefits for patients of reducing medication (e.g. quality of life) or a reduction in costs. When choosing outcome measures for evaluation, it is important to consider unintended negative consequences, as discussed in Chapter 7. For example, removing a screening test may be necessary, but could lead to a decrease in patients' trust in the healthcare system and subsequently to poorer engagement in care and missed opportunities for detecting other diseases (Norton and Chambers 2020). Perceptions of de-implementation interventions may be different in different groups, including minority groups due, for example, to historical health disparities, and this should be considered and measured if possible (Prusaczyk et al. 2020).

## TYPES OF EVALUATIONS

To address whether a de-implementation intervention led to the reduction or removal of unsafe or ineffective medical practices, you should think about the purpose of your evaluation and what resources are available to conduct it. Typically, there are two broad evaluation methods that you may consider: randomised and non-randomised evaluations. Your choice may depend on the certainty you want about the results and available resources. Programme evaluation and monitoring may assess whether an intervention was *associated* with reductions in low-value care in your context and you may be willing to accept a lower level of certainty about whether your intervention *caused* the change. In this case, a less rigorous (often non-randomised) method can be adopted. Research evaluations usually require greater certainty about whether your intervention *caused* any reductions in low-value care and typically use more rigorous (preferably randomised) methods. In this chapter, we will provide a high-level summary of evaluation designs; readers wanting more detail should consult key methodological references (Donner and Klar 2000; Kahan et al. 2022a; Kahan 2013; Kahan et al. 2022b; Grimshaw et al. 2000; Hemming and Taljaard 2020).

## Randomised Evaluations

Randomised evaluations, in their simplest form, are comparable to tossing a coin to decide which individuals will be in the de-implementation intervention group and which ones will be in the control group, receiving no, or a competing, intervention. Randomisation allows an unbiased, fair comparison between the two groups, because the two groups are likely to be similar in everything except whether they receive the intervention or not. A randomised evaluation is less likely to suffer from bias but can take more time or resources to conduct. The simplest randomised evaluations randomise individuals such as patients. More often, de-implementation interventions are aimed at groups of healthcare professionals known as *clusters*, such as family practices or hospitals. These interventions should be evaluated using *cluster randomised trials* where clusters are randomised to either intervention or control. When planning a cluster randomised trial, it is important to involve a statistician to calculate the number of clusters needed and undertake the analyses (van Smeden 2022). There are different types of cluster trials. In Box 10.1, we describe three commonly used designs: the parallel arm cluster trial, the factorial trial, and the stepped wedge design.

### Box 10.1   Three Types of Cluster Randomised Trials

#### Parallel Arm Cluster Randomised Trials

Comparing groups can be done using a design called parallel arm. If the comparison involves two groups, it is called a two-arm parallel trial. If it involves more than two groups, it is a multi-arm parallel trial. This design tends to be straightforward to implement and analyse but might be less efficient statistically than alternative designs like factorial or stepped wedge (i.e. it might need more clusters or participants).

The Effective Feedback to Improve Primary Care Prescribing Safety (EFIPPS) trial (Guthrie et al. 2016) is an example of this. EFIPPS was a three-arm cluster *randomised controlled trial* that compared providing data feedback and a behavioural change intervention with usual care to improve primary care prescribing safety. Primary care practices were randomised to: usual care; usual care plus feedback on practice's high-risk prescribing; or usual care plus the same feedback incorporating a behavioural change component. The authors chose cluster randomisation because feedback of high-risk prescribing data was done at practice level.

### Factorial Trials

If you have an interest in evaluating two separate interventions delivered simultaneously, then you may consider a factorial trial. The advantage is that you test the interventions at the same time and in the same group of clusters or participants (Kahan 2013). This assumes that the interventions do not interact and are independent from each other (Kahan et al. 2022b).

NEXUS (Eccles et al. 2001) was a *two-by-two factorial trial*, which aimed to reduce GP requests for radiological tests. The researchers were interested in evaluating the impact of audit and feedback with and without educational reminder messages. Practices were randomised into one of four groups: (i) audit and feedback only, (ii) educational reminder messages only, (iii) audit and feedback + educational reminder messages, and (iv) control (guideline alone). This allowed them to test those interventions simultaneously but recruiting a sample size equivalent to a parallel arm trial that only tests a single intervention.

**Stepped Wedge Designs**

Stepped wedge designs are useful when all clusters must receive the intervention at some point for logistical or political reasons (Prost et al. 2015). In this design, each cluster 'turns on' the intervention at a specific randomly allocated time. At the start of the trial, no cluster is receiving the intervention. At the end, all clusters received the intervention (Hemming et al. 2015). This can be challenging to run from a logistical perspective (Dreischulte et al. 2013).

An example is a *stepped-wedge cluster randomised trial* among patients on 12 acute medical or surgical hospital wards (Haines et al. 2017). It was focused on de-implementing weekend allied health services. This service was incrementally removed from participating wards each calendar month, in a random order. The analyses adjusted for naturally occurring change over time.

## Non-Randomised Evaluations

In non-randomised evaluations, the assignment of the intervention is made by non-random means. For example, individuals, practices, or wards sign up to take part in a de-implementation intervention (self-selection) or managers or legislators choose which units will receive the intervention (administrator selection). In these evaluations, you may still have control over some features, such as selecting and scheduling when outcomes are measured, deciding what control groups are included, or scheduling delivery of interventions (Shadish et al. 2002). Non-randomised evaluations provide less compelling support than randomised evaluations about whether the intervention caused a change in outcomes. This is because factors such as time and self-selection to receive the intervention may play a role in the observed effect of the intervention.

Therefore, alternative explanations to the observed effects of the intervention (or lack of) should be considered. Two popular types of non-randomised evaluations are: before and after and interrupted time-series (ITS) evaluations. These evaluations are explained in Box 10.2.

## Box 10.2   Two Types of Non-randomised Trials

### Before and After Evaluations

These designs assess whether the intervention was successful by looking at data before and after the intervention was implemented. However, they are likely to be biased because of possible time trends in practice or due to other events occurring at the same time as the intervention. Controlled before and after evaluations include a group of similar units (e.g. family practices or hospitals) not undertaking the intervention used as the control or comparator to the intervention practices. Intervention and control units' data are compared after the intervention is implemented, and any differences found are attributed to the intervention. You may find it difficult to recruit control units in your setting; and the effect of time can still be hard to measure. If the control units are not comparable to the intervention arm units, then your results might be biased. Before and after evaluations are popular because they are relatively easy to conduct, but your ability to draw robust conclusions about cause–effect is limited.

An example of a *before and after study* evaluated a knowledge transfer and exchange intervention designed to de-implement 'in-house' occupational therapy tools and replace them with evidence-based tools in homecare services in Quebec (Canada) (Guay et al. 2019). Data were collected in 94 health and social services centres providing homecare services before and after the intervention. At the end, de-implementation of 'in-house' tools and their replacement with evidence-based tools was measured.

**Interrupted Time Series**

This is a variation on a before and after evaluation, involving collecting data consistently at multiple and equally spaced time points before and after an 'interruption', in your case the de-implementation intervention (Grimshaw et al. 2000). This implies that, when designing an ITS evaluation, you need to consider when and how often you can measure data. The main objective of an ITS is to assess whether the data pattern observed post-intervention is different to that observed pre-intervention. These analyses are the most robust to assess an intervention when randomised trials are not feasible (Bernal et al. 2017). Adding a control group or starting the intervention at different times can strengthen the design (Shadish et al. 2002). ITS are best used to evaluate interventions introduced at a clearly defined point in time. The ITS design without a control group is not protected against the effects of other events occurring at the same time as the study intervention (Kontopantelis et al. 2015).

An example of an *ITS study* was the reduce inappropriate use of intravenous and urinary catheters (RICAT) study (Laan et al. 2020). It was a multicentre study in seven hospitals, without a control group. Data on catheter use were collected every two weeks during the baseline period (seven months) and post-intervention period (seven months), which were separated by a five-month intervention period. The data before and after the intervention were compared using an ITS analysis. The primary outcome was percentage of catheters used inappropriately.

## SELECTING THE MOST APPROPRIATE EVALUATION METHOD

The choice of the most appropriate evaluation method is challenging. Key considerations presented in Figure 10.1 include:

- *Is randomisation possible?*
  Randomisation might not be possible due to several reasons including: it is not acceptable to randomise the intervention;

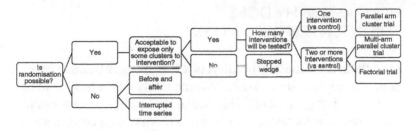

**FIGURE 10.1** Selecting the most appropriate evaluation method.
*Source*: Adapted from Rogers van Katwyk (2020).

it is too difficult to implement randomisation in practice because the evaluators have little control over when or who will receive the intervention; or the number of clusters is not enough to randomise. If fewer than six to eight clusters are available, then cluster randomised evaluations are not recommended (Donner and Klar 2000; Leyrat et al. 2018; Barker et al. 2017). The trade-off is that even though non-randomised evaluations require a small number of units (e.g. clinical practices or hospitals), they usually require measurements in different, and multiple intervals. Most de-implementation evaluations do not use a randomised design: more than 80% of the de-implementation articles in a recent review used a before and after evaluation without a control group (Cliff et al. 2021).

- *Is it acceptable to expose only some clusters to the intervention?*

  In some instances, for example for political reasons, it may be unacceptable to expose only some clusters to the intervention. If that is the case, a stepped wedge design where all clusters eventually get the intervention is the preferred option when randomisation is possible.

- *How many interventions will be tested?*

  This will help determine the type of evaluation you should use. For example, factorial experiments or multi-arm designs are only appropriate when two or more (active) interventions will be compared to a control.

## HOW AND WHY DOES THE INTERVENTION WORK?

In addition to evaluating the effect of a de-implementation interven-tion, you might want to know how the intervention has led to the achieved effect (or lack of). This can be studied in a process evalua-tion. Process evaluations aim to explain what happened, such as which part of the intervention was most successful and why, or why some clusters have greater improvement than others. This can be useful for (i) improving the intervention(s) in the participating clus-ters; (ii) refining the intervention(s) so that they are more likely to be adopted successfully in other clusters; and (iii) generating knowledge on the process of de-implementing low-value care.

There are multiple guides to inform process evaluations (Saunders et al. 2005; Grant et al. 2013), for example, the UK Medical Research Council (MRC) guide (see Figure 10.2) describes three key aspects that can be considered in a process evaluation: implementation, mechanism, and contextual. These aspects can be measured using different methods such as surveys, interviews, electronic health record data, or observations. In Box 10.3, we describe these three aspects.

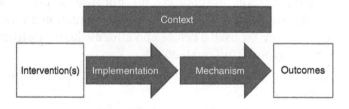

**FIGURE 10.2**   The MRC process evaluation framework. *Source*: Moore, 2015/BMJ Publishing/CC BY 4.0.

### Box 10.3   Three Key Aspects of a Process Evaluation

#### Implementation

This aspect focuses on the actual delivery of the intervention and whether it is done according to what was originally planned as deviations might have major influences on the intended effect. Example: the de-implementation strategy to reduce inappropriate intravenous and urinary catheters (see Box 10.2 [Laan et al. 2020]) also included patient leaflets. These aimed to educate patients on the indications for catheters, and patients were asked to alert their nurse or doctor when they suspected that their catheter could be removed. However, the process evaluation of this study showed that many nurses did not hand out the leaflets to patients, because they thought the leaflets were too difficult for patients to understand or they did not agree with their content. When most patients are not exposed to the leaflet, its full effect cannot be evaluated.

The implementation process can be evaluated by measuring the fidelity (whether the intervention was delivered as intended), dose (the quantity of intervention implemented), and reach (to what extent the intended audience encounters the intervention) of the intervention.

## Mechanism

Mechanisms through which interventions bring change can be complex, but studying them can provide significant insight in how the intervention has worked and why (Grimshaw et al. 2007). Example: the DRAM study evaluated the use of audit and feedback and education messages to reduce unnecessary laboratory testing by GPs in Scotland (Thomas et al. 2006). The authors hypothesised that the interventions would work by strengthening intentions to order fewer tests by increasing attitudes and social norms. A formal mediation analysis demonstrated that the intervention partially worked through these mechanisms (Ramsay et al. 2010).

Mechanistic process evaluations can also help detect unanticipated consequences. Example: several GP practices in the Netherlands received education on vitamin D and B12 testing, aiming to reduce unnecessary testing (van Vugt et al. 2021). A second set of GP practices also received additional educational materials for patients: a video and leaflets available in waiting rooms. After the intervention, the process evaluation took place using interviews with GPs and patients. This showed that the waiting room materials prompted several patients to ask for a vitamin test, even though they had not planned on asking this when they scheduled an appointment. This information can be used to further improve the intervention. In this case, one might consider to only use the video and leaflet when patients have already asked for a vitamin D or B12 test instead of presenting them in the waiting room.

### Context

Contextual factors include all external factors that may affect the implementation, the mechanism of impact, and the outcomes. For every de-implementation intervention, different contextual factors may play a role, depending on the type of low-value care practice, the target audience of the intervention, and societal and political situation. Example: a de-implementation study aimed to reduce unnecessary diagnostic testing on internal medicine departments using a multifaceted intervention (Bindraban et al. 2019). A survey amongst clinicians was used to evaluate the process. They found several barriers to the interventions, such as a rapid turnover of junior physicians and a lack of time to participate in the project. An enabling factor was the enthusiasm of colleagues. With this knowledge, the intervention was improved by incorporating education on (un)necessary diagnostic testing in the introduction programme for new junior physicians.

## DOES THE INTERVENTION OFFER GOOD VALUE FOR MONEY?

Value for money evaluation, usually named economic evaluation, is a systematic framework concerned with assessing the outcomes and costs arising from interventions (Drummond et al. 2015).

In de-implementation, economic evaluation involves comparing the costs of various de-implementation interventions and identifying the most efficient method given scarce healthcare resources. The viewpoint selected for the evaluation, either a patient, a hospital, or a third-party payer, determines the type of costs and the extent to which they are included. This will inform the decision of whether the strategy is or is not good value for money. Proposed frameworks for economic evaluation for implementation science have been described elsewhere (Eisman et al. 2020; Severens et al. 2020; Reeves et al. 2019).

Economic evaluation can be performed using person-level and decision modelling approaches. Person-level economic evaluation is often conducted alongside (randomised) clinical trials, which may have a short follow-up duration and may not reflect the real world of clinical practice. Some economic evaluations are conducted based on health administrative data or electronic medical records; however, these evaluations might be biased and require advanced statistical analyses. Decision modelling has been increasingly used for economic evaluations because it allows researchers to reflect on possible consequences of alternative strategies being evaluated, integrate multiple sources of data such as clinical trials and administrative data, and assess the uncertainty about the economic evaluation results.

## KEY POINTS

- Evaluating your de-implementation intervention will tell you whether it has delivered what it intended to deliver, and whether it avoided unintended negative consequences.
- A rigorous evaluation can be a good way to reassure colleagues of the importance of further reducing the low-value care practice and as a base of scaling the intervention.
- Understanding the implementation, mechanism, and context of your intervention, and its cost-effectiveness are important to gain the understanding of how and why your intervention has worked and whether it is feasible to implement it in the health system.

# REFERENCES

Barker, D., D'Este, C., Campbell, M.J. et al. (2017). Minimum number of clusters and comparison of analysis methods for cross sectional stepped wedge cluster randomised trials with binary outcomes: a simulation study. *Trials* 18: 1–11.

Bernal, J.L., Cummins, S., and Gasparrini, A. (2017). Interrupted time series regression for the evaluation of public health interventions: a tutorial. *International Journal of Epidemiology* 46: 348–355.

Bindraban, R.S., van Beneden, M., Kramer, M.H. et al. (2019). Association of a multifaceted intervention with ordering of unnecessary laboratory tests among caregivers in internal medicine departments. *JAMA Network Open* 2: e197577–e197577.

Born, K., Patey, A., Grimshaw, J. et al. (2018). Letter in response to: "CJEM debate series: # ChoosingWisely – the Choosing Wisely campaign will not impact physician behaviour and choices". *Canadian Journal of Emergency Medicine* 20: 1–1.

Cliff, B.Q., Avancena, A.L., Hirth, R.A. et al. (2021). The impact of Choosing Wisely interventions on low-value medical services: a systematic review. *The Milbank Quarterly* 99: 1024–1058.

Donner, A. and Klar, N. (2000). *Design and Analysis of Cluster Randomization Trials in Health Research*. Arnold Publishers.

Dreischulte, T., Grant, A., Donnan, P. et al. (2013). Pro's and con's of the stepped wedge design in cluster randomised trials of quality improvement interventions: two current examples. *Trials* 14: 1–1.

Drummond, M.F., Sculpher, M.J., Claxton, K. et al. (2015). *Methods for the Economic Evaluation of Health Care Programmes*. Oxford University Press.

Eccles, M., Steen, N., Grimshaw, J. et al. (2001). Effect of audit and feedback, and reminder messages on primary-care radiology referrals: a randomised trial. *The Lancet* 357: 1406–1409.

Eisman, A.B., Kilbourne, A.M., Dopp, A.R. et al. (2020). Economic evaluation in implementation science: making the business case for implementation strategies. *Psychiatry Research* 283: 112433.

Grant, A., Treweek, S., Dreischulte, T. et al. (2013). Process evaluations for cluster-randomised trials of complex interventions: a proposed framework for design and reporting. *Trials* 14: 1–10.

Grimshaw, J., Campbell, M., Eccles, M. et al. (2000). Experimental and quasi-experimental designs for evaluating guideline implementation strategies. *Family Practice* 17: S11–S16.

Grimshaw, J.M., Zwarenstein, M., Tetroe, J.M. et al. (2007). Looking inside the black box: a theory-based process evaluation alongside a randomised controlled trial of printed educational materials (the Ontario printed educational message, OPEM) to improve referral and prescribing practices in primary care in Ontario, Canada. *Implementation Science* 2: 1–8.

Grimshaw, J.M., Patey, A.M., Kirkham, K.R. et al. (2020). De-implementing wisely: developing the evidence base to reduce low-value care. *BMJ Quality and Safety* https://doi.org/10.1136/bmjqs-2019-010060.

Guay, M., Ruest, M., and Contandriopoulos, D. (2019). Deimplementing untested practices in homecare services: a preobservational-postobservational design. *Occupational Therapy International*, 2019.

Guthrie, B., Kavanagh, K., Robertson, C. et al. (2016). Data feedback and behavioural change intervention to improve primary care prescribing safety (EFIPPS): multicentre, three arm, cluster randomised controlled trial. *British Medical Journal* 354: i4079.

Haines, T.P., Bowles, K.-A., Mitchell, D. et al. (2017). Impact of disinvestment from weekend allied health services across acute medical and surgical wards: 2 stepped-wedge cluster randomised controlled trials. *PLoS Medicine* 14: e1002412.

Hemming, K. and Taljaard, M. (2020). Reflection on modern methods: when is a stepped-wedge cluster randomized trial a good study design choice? *International Journal of Epidemiology* 49: 1043–1052.

Hemming, K., Haines, T.P., Chilton, P.J. et al. (2015). The stepped wedge cluster randomised trial: rationale, design, analysis, and reporting. *BMJ* 350: h391.

Kahan, B.C. (2013). Bias in randomised factorial trials. *Statistics in Medicine* 32: 4540–4549.

Kahan, B.C., Li, F., Copas, A.J. et al. (2022a). Estimands in cluster-randomized trials: choosing analyses that answer the right question. *International Journal of Epidemiology* 52: 107–118.

Kahan, B.C., Morris, T.P., Goulão, B. et al. (2022b). Estimands for factorial trials. *Statistics in Medicine* 41: 4299–4310.

Kontopantelis, E., Doran, T., Springate, D.A. et al. (2015). Regression based quasi-experimental approach when randomisation is not an option: interrupted time series analysis. *BMJ* 350: h2750.

Laan, B.J., Maaskant, J.M., Spijkerman, I.J.B. et al. (2020). De-implementation strategy to reduce inappropriate use of intravenous and urinary catheters (RICAT): a multicentre, prospective, interrupted time-series and before and after study. *Lancet Infectious Diseases* 20: 864–872.

Leyrat, C., Morgan, K.E., Leurent, B. et al. (2018). Cluster randomized trials with a small number of clusters: which analyses should be used? *International Journal of Epidemiology* 47: 321–331.

Moore, G.F., Audrey, S., Barker, M. et al. (2015). Process evaluation of complex interventions: Medical Research Council guidance. *BMJ* 350: h1258.

Norton, W.E. and Chambers, D.A. (2020). Unpacking the complexities of de-implementing inappropriate health interventions. *Implementation Science* 15: 1–7.

Prost, A., Binik, A., Abubakar, I. et al. (2015). Logistic, ethical, and political dimensions of stepped wedge trials: critical review and case studies. *Trials* 16: 1–11.

Prusaczyk, B., Swindle, T., and Curran, G. (2020). Defining and conceptualizing outcomes for de-implementation: key distinctions from implementation outcomes. *Implementation Science Communications* 1: 1–10.

Ramsay, C.R., Thomas, R.E., Croal, B.L. et al. (2010). Using the theory of planned behaviour as a process evaluation tool in randomised trials of knowledge translation strategies: a case study from UK primary care. *Implementation Science* 5: 1–9.

Reeves, P., Edmunds, K., Searles, A. et al. (2019). Economic evaluations of public health implementation-interventions: a systematic review and guideline for practice. *Public Health* 169: 101–113.

Rogers Van Katwyk, S., Hoffman, S., Mendelson, M. et al. (2020). Strengthening the science of addressing antimicrobial resistance: a framework for planning, conducting and disseminating antimicrobial resistance intervention research. *Health Research Policy and Systems* 18: 1–13.

Saunders, R.P., Evans, M.H., and Joshi, P. (2005). Developing a process-evaluation plan for assessing health promotion program implementation: a how-to guide. *Health Promotion Practice* 6: 134–147.

Severens, J.L., Hoomans, T., Adang, E. et al. (2020). Economic evaluation of implementation strategies. In: *Improving Patient Care: The Implementation of Change in Health Care* (ed. M. Wensing, R. Grol, and J. Grimshaw), 389–408. http://doi.org/10.1002/9781119488620.ch23

Shadish, W.R., Cook, T.D., and Campbell, D.T. (2002). *Experimental and Quasi-Experimental Designs for Generalized Causal Inference.* Houghton, Mifflin and Company.

van Smeden, M. (2022). A very short list of common pitfalls in research design, Data Analysis, and Reporting. *PRiMER* 6: 26.

Thomas, R.E., Croal, B.L., Ramsay, C. et al. (2006). Effect of enhanced feedback and brief educational reminder messages on laboratory test requesting in primary care: a cluster randomised trial. *The Lancet* 367: 1990–1996.

van Vugt, S., de Schepper, E., van Delft, S. et al. (2021). Effectiveness of professional and patient-oriented strategies in reducing vitamin D and B12 test ordering in primary care: a cluster randomised intervention study. *British Journal of General Practice Open* 5.

# Preserving Results and Spreading Interventions: Phase 4

Simone van Dulmen, Daniëlle Kroon, and Tijn Kool

*Department of IQ Healthcare, Radboud University Medical Center, Radboud Institute for Health Sciences, Nijmegen, The Netherlands*

## WHY ARE SUSTAINABILITY AND SPREAD SO IMPORTANT?

De-implementation is critical for ensuring long-term quality and affordability of healthcare. Once the process of (de-)implementation is completed, there is often a tendency to relapse into old routines (Grol and Grimshaw 2003). Sustainability of behaviour change is a persistent challenge, and experts have prioritised it as one of the most significant translational research problems of our time (Proctor et al. 2015). De-implementation efforts would be a waste of resources if intervention successes are unintentionally reversed after the end of a project. Moreover, the consequences are not just financial but may also result in suboptimal care, cause frustration, and diminish the support for future healthcare

*How to Reduce Overuse in Healthcare: A Practical Guide*, First Edition.
Edited by Tijn Kool, Andrea M. Patey, Simone van Dulmen, and Jeremy M. Grimshaw.
© 2024 John Wiley & Sons Ltd. Published 2024 by John Wiley & Sons Ltd.

improvement initiatives. Therefore, it is important that de-implementation successes are sustained in the long term. Even when initial de-implementation efforts are successful, it is not always possible to maintain the original interventions. This may be due to changes in priorities, resource availability, or other contextual factors. Fortunately, sustainability of the results does not always require a continuation of the initial de-implementation strategy. Therefore, we focus on the sustainability of the effects rather than the intervention itself. Understanding this process and determining how to foster the maintenance of behaviour change to yield desired health outcomes is at least as important as understanding how to implement interventions in the first place. And this process can help to understand, predict, and increase the chances of long-term sustainability.

Besides sustained effects within an organisation, for widescale effects, the intervention should also be implemented in other organisations. The spread of interventions within and between hospitals will be perceived as further confirmation of its effectiveness and will increase the intention to sustain the results in accordance with the implemented programmes (Ament et al. 2017). Spreading the project to other organisations may face other challenges, as the local context is often different.

## WHAT IS SUSTAINABILITY?

Many terms have been used to describe sustainability, such as 'continuation', 'maintenance', 'durability', 'adoption', 'embedding', and 'institutionalisation', among others (Shediac-Rizkallah and Bone 1998; Scheirer et al. 2008). We define the sustainability of an intervention as the degree in which an intervention delivers its intended benefits after the de-implementation phase has ended. For patients, sustainability could be realised when patients do not still receive low-value care in the future. For an organisation, sustainability is about whether, in the long term, its healthcare professionals are aware of high-value care practices and do not fall back into old patterns of providing low-value care.

In previous chapters, we have seen that getting sustainable results is a challenge. Behavioural change by breaking through routines and habits demands a tailor-made strategy. Still, this does not guarantee that any changes will persist. If you want to explain why the intervention is sustainable or not, an evaluation of the processes and factors that may facilitate or hinder the continuation of effect of the intervention is needed (Chapter 10). There have been several studies investigating the sustainability of the effects (Shelton et al. 2018; Wiltsey Stirman et al. 2012). Studies have emphasised the importance of starting to develop specific sustainability strategies throughout the planning phase of an intervention (Pluye et al. 2004). Effective sustainment strategies for de-implementation interventions are not well reported (Hailemariam et al. 2019). There is increasing research about the effects of de-implementation; however, most of these studies do not investigate whether the effects of the interventions remain over a longer period (Heus et al. 2023).

## FACTORS INFLUENCING SUSTAINED CHANGE

The UK National Health Service (NHS) has developed a model that identifies all relevant factors to make interventions sustainable, the NHS Sustainability Model. The model includes nine factors about the process, staff, and organisation that are important to realise sustainability (see Figure 11.1).

### Factors Related to the Process

1. The intervention should, in addition to helping patients, improve the process and have benefits beyond helping patients such as advantage for staff and a more efficient process.

   Healthcare professionals should be encouraged to keep the de-implementation intervention alive. For example, by using the electronic health records (EHRs) for

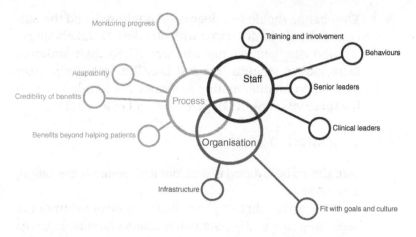

**FIGURE 11.1** Factors on the process, staff, and organisation related to sustainability. *Source*: Sustainability Model and Guide. Reproduced with the permission of Dr. Maher (Lynne Maher and Evan 2010).

automatic actions. In Dutch hospitals, this was done for dermatologists to provide tailor-made patient information automatically from the electronic patient record. This helped to sustain the restriction of follow-up visits after basal cell carcinoma (van Egmond et al. 2022).

2. Benefits should be clear for everyone, and evidence that it works is needed.

   Guidelines or lists from professional societies, such as produced in the Choosing Wisely campaigns, can support the strength of the evidence. Moreover, local evidence from performance evaluation and monitoring or generalisable evidence from research evaluations may be helpful.

3. The change should not depend on specific people or resources and should fulfil ongoing needs.

   Leaders are important, but they should aim at changing infrastructure and culture structurally. It might help, for example, to change the way blood tests are ordered in the electronic patient record if the aim is to reduce laboratory testing.

4. The change should be adequately monitored, and the outcomes should be discussed with all relevant stakeholders.

Showing general practitioners (GPs) their ordering behaviour of vitamin B12 and D will help to keep them focused on an intervention to reduce the number of testing these vitamins in GP practice (Vugt et al. 2021).

## Factors Related to Staff

1. Staff should be involved in development, de-implementation, and training.

It is crucial that staff members are involved from the beginning to identify potential barriers and enablers (see Chapter 8) and use their knowledge and experience to help design the de-implementation intervention (see Chapter 9). You can organise focus groups or interviews to identify their thoughts on the planned change.

2. The behaviours of the staff towards sustaining the change should be clear.

It should be very clear whether the staff is concerned about the effects of the intervention. If there are any concerns, these should be discussed and addressed, if possible. If healthcare professionals are concerned that a specific intervention takes too much time, it is important to arrange enough support and to show staff that they will be facilitated.

3. Senior and clinical leaders should be engaged.

Senior staff members can be the talking heads of your strategy. Their seniority can convince peers and residents about the importance of that strategy. They can be an important part of your communication strategy.

## Factors Related to the Organisation

1. The change should fit the organisational strategy and culture.

It is important to show that the intervention is aligned with existing organisational culture. Does it help to fulfil the organisational goals? Does the intervention fit in the

plans that have been made by the organisation? If a hospital has a strategic vision that networks are essential, it might help that the planned de-implementation intervention facilitates cooperation.
2. The infrastructure should facilitate the change.

The staff should be trained and competent in the new way of working. There should be enough facilities and equipment to support the new process. And the organisational policies and procedures should support the new way of working. If you want to reduce the number of expensive bandages on the emergency department, those bandages should not be for the taking on the bandage car but only on request.

## HOW CAN YOU FACILITATE SUSTAINABILITY?

There are several strategies that are crucial to facilitate sustainability. By using these strategies, healthcare professionals better understand the sense and value of the intervention and the impact of it. They will help grow shared motivation (Flynn et al. 2021). It is crucial to take these strategies into account when designing the intervention to increase the change of getting sustainable effects. We describe the strategies with an example of reducing inappropriate urinary and intravenous catheters:

– Organise a regular *learning collaborative*
  Many de-implementation initiatives start on a project basis. When working on a project basis, there is a risk that those involved will lose their attention when the project is finished. To create lasting awareness, you can plan several meetings with relevant healthcare professionals of your own organisation or from several organisations and discuss the specific de-implementation intervention and its results. This motivates healthcare professionals and might inspire them to improve the intervention. For example, nurses from different departments or hospitals can discuss their activities in reducing inappropriate urinary and intravasal catheters

(Laan et al. 2020). They can share their experiences, successes, and challenges and present their data to each other.

– Give regular *audit and feedback*

By informing the relevant healthcare professionals about the progress they made in attaining the desired outcomes, for example, the reduction of inappropriate catheters, you can motivate nurses of the abovementioned learning collaborative to stay focused on the appropriate indication for catheters. Comparative feedback may motivate healthcare professionals to attain at least comparable results as their colleagues (Laan et al. 2020).

– Organise *informal leadership*

You can ask specific healthcare professionals that are informal clinical leaders to keep on asking whether the catheters have the appropriate indication and keep on emphasising the importance of attention to the indication for a catheter.

– Draw attention by *patient stories*

You can emphasise the importance of focus on the intervention by talking about patients who were harmed by not paying attention to the indication. You might discuss the case of a patient that got a urinary sepsis after having a urinary catheter for too long.

– *Embedded* strategies *in daily practices*

The change should no longer be experienced as extra, but as a standard procedure. In reducing unnecessary urinary catheters, it might help introducing a smart phrase in the electronic patient record that asks the physician and nurse during rounds whether the indication for the catheter is still valid.

## ASSESSING SUSTAINABILITY

Sustainability can be assessed in different ways. One approach is to continue measuring (patient relevant) outcomes from the original de-implementation project. Other potential sustainability measures include: (i) continued awareness of healthcare professionals of the low-value care practice; (ii) maintaining community-level partnerships and community capacity for collaboration; (iii) maintaining organisational practices, procedures, and policies started during the de-implementation programme (institutionalisation); or (iv) continuing the programme activities or core elements of the original intervention (Shelton et al. 2018).

## SUSTAINABILITY AND CULTURE

The sustainability of a de-implementation intervention can be facilitated or inhibited by the organisation's culture. Organisational culture pertains to multiple shared characteristics among people within the same organisation including: beliefs, values, norms of behaviour, routines, traditions, sense-making, etc. (Parmelli et al. 2011). Cultural elements that facilitate the (de)implementation itself and its sustainability are as follows:

- A supportive culture entails positive signalling and leadership. For example, a message that aligns low-value care de-implementation with the broader organisational mission can create a sense of urgency by stressing that unnecessary services are a barrier to high-quality, affordable, and equitable care.
- Couching low-value care within broader priorities to achieve value-based care and outcomes. This might help those within the organisation envision a grander purpose of de-implementation, instead of silo initiatives focused on stopping or reducing one specific aspect of care (Sorenson and Japinga 2022).
- Facilitating healthcare provider-driven initiatives. Organisations can contribute to the success of implementation by supporting healthcare professional initiated interventions, given their clinical expertise, direct interaction in care delivery, and views that modification of their beliefs and behaviour is essential for change. There should be a culture

of trust, open communication, and safety in order to learn from each other (Parchman et al. 2017).

- Prioritising and supporting innovation. This could be facilitated by annual budgets or funds, as well as offering opportunities to educate peers and care teams on the harms of low-value care to patients, professionals, and organisational reputation, and to coordinate and lead de-implementation projects.
- Facilitating data collection and measurement tools. Given the central role of data in identifying and monitoring low-value care use, organisations should facilitate data collection and measurement tools, and strategies to leverage existing tools, such as performance dashboards, report cards, clinical decision supports, and other technology (e.g. telehealth, EHRs, iPads, or cell phones).

## SPREADING SUCCESSFUL DE-IMPLEMENTATION INTERVENTIONS

Successful interventions should not only be sustainable but should also be scaled to other organisations and healthcare providers. Many de-implementation projects start locally, and the spread of these interventions rarely occurs spontaneously.

The challenge of spreading interventions is widely acknowledged. Everett Rogers first introduced his Diffusion of Innovations Theory in 1962, and it is applied in many fields, including healthcare. For this reason, the literature mainly focuses on the spread of innovations rather than de-implementation interventions. Although there are several similarities, de-implementation interventions are not equivalent to innovations. These differences are also relevant for the dissemination process. For example, we know that the spread of interventions is facilitated if the intervention is compatible with the values of adopters. Innovations create additional treatment options. This naturally fits with the values of healthcare professionals because they are trained to do something for their patients (Haas et al. 2012; Rosenbaum and Lamas 2012;

Lakhani et al. 2016). On the other hand, de-implementation interventions are often aiming at 'not doing', which could seem to undermine professional integrity (Hofmann 2021). This suggests that de-implementation requires more attention and perhaps different approaches to meet the values of healthcare professionals. This starts with the design of the de-implementation intervention. One should be aware of the fact that it asks for a different approach to convince potential adopters to implement the intervention. There are four main topics that need to be addressed in designing a scale-up project: the scaling strategy, the de-implementation intervention, the external context, and the adopters.

## Scaling Strategy

Someone or a team needs to be responsible for the scale-up project. This person/team has several tasks: to evaluate, tailor and adapt the de-implementation intervention to the new context, find ways to reach adopters and support them in implementing the intervention, and to make use of existing incentives or create new ones. These tasks require extended knowledge about the original intervention and also about the context in which the intervention will be scaled. The innovators are probably in the best position to assess and adjust the de-implementation intervention, and to support adopters with the implementation. Therefore, it is essential to partner with them in a scale-up project. They know the do's and don'ts of the intervention, so they are the ones who can support and advise the local adopters in implementing it the best way possible. Consider also partnering with organisations that are well-known and have a wide reach among potential adopters. This will facilitate reaching adopters and convincing them to implement the intervention. Other ways of reaching adopters are through professional and social networks. For example, you can ask every involved professional to invite colleagues in other organisations to learn more about the intervention. Or look for organisations with a network that can easily communicate with potential adopters and ask them if they are willing to publish a news item on the intervention.

The success of multi-centre de-implementation interventions depends on the support and effort of the coordinating (research) team. Interaction between participants of different sites is often motivating, stimulating, and inspiring. It is important to also create this kind of interaction in a scale-up project. Start, for example, a learning collaboration, as mentioned earlier above for the sustainability. This networking brings all healthcare professionals together and enable them to discuss difficulties and share successes.

## De-Implementation Intervention

The potential adopters need to be convinced about the advantage of the de-implementation intervention. This requires strong evidence that the clinical practice is of low-value and that the de-implementation intervention is successful.

The scale-up team needs to critically review the de-implementation intervention before the start of the actual project. Because at this point, you can still improve the feasibility of the intervention. There are a several aspects to consider regarding the feasibility. First, the intervention should be compatible with the values and beliefs of the adopters. The local context may differ between hospitals or other healthcare organisations. Therefore, the adopters should be able to adjust the intervention to meet the local needs and fit into setting. This will not only promote the compatibility, but also enables the local teams to redesign the de-implementation intervention as required. This redesign can help by making the adopters feel like they create their own intervention. The feasibility is also improved if the effects of the de-implementation interventions are easy to monitor, because observable change helps motivate the adopters to continue the project. Moreover, negative side effects or stagnation can be identified, and the local team can act upon such results. The last aspect is the complexity of the de-implementation intervention. The intervention should preferably be simple, or otherwise divided in several steps. The adopters can start small and expand the intervention at their convenience.

## Adopters or Adopting Organisation

De-implementation interventions will only be adopted by healthcare professionals who feel the need to change. Therefore, the scale-up team needs to identify those healthcare professionals who recognise the negative effects of particular low-value care and who are willing to change their way of working. Sometimes the adopters of a disseminated intervention are not the same as initial project leaders. For example, a Dutch de-implementation project to reduce the inappropriate use of intravenous catheters and urine catheters was originally aimed at residents and internists (Laan et al. 2020). But, during the dissemination, there was more enthusiasm for the project and willingness to change by nurses than by clinicians. The focus was changed to nurses, and many more hospitals with enthusiastic nurses adopted the project.

## External Context

The external context or environment, in which the intervention will be spread, should contain incentives to use it. Incentives are drivers of interventions on top of the advantage of the intervention. Examples of incentives are a clinical guideline stating that a practice is of low value, accreditation for education on low-value care, and scientific opportunities for the de-implementation project. However, incentives for de-implementation are often lacking, while incentives to provide low-value care are strongly present. For example, providing low-value care can be profitable for healthcare providers, and de-implementation of these practices could result in a financial disadvantage. Therefore, to ease the spread of de-implementation interventions, the incentives to provide low-value care should be removed, and incentives for de-implementation need to be created.

It may seem that healthcare professionals are not able to create incentives. However, in the past decade, we have witnessed how the de-implementation lobby arose. This lobby created the current societal demand for de-implementation. Healthcare professionals, healthcare insurers, politicians, and citizens are more and more aware of the risks of low-value care and are demanding a change.

## KEY POINTS

- Sustainability of the result of interventions is challenging and requires continuous effort after the de-implementation phase and implementation of key elements in daily practice.
- Sustainability and spread of the results are interrelated; sustained results might facilitate further spreading activities
- Scaling does not occur spontaneously, but it requires: a scaling team with a strategy to raise awareness and support of adopters; a feasible intervention with strong evidence and that can be modified by local teams; adopters who feel the need for change; and an external context with incentives to de-implement low-value care.

## REFERENCES

Ament, S.M.C., Gillissen, F., Moser, A. et al. (2017). Factors associated with sustainability of 2 quality improvement programs after achieving early implementation success. A qualitative case study. *Journal of Evaluation in Clinical Practice* 23: 1135–1143.

Flynn, R., Mrklas, K., Campbell, A. et al. (2021). Contextual factors and mechanisms that influence sustainability: a realist evaluation of two scaled, multi-component interventions. *BMC Health Services Research* 21: 1194.

Grol, R. and Grimshaw, J. (2003). From best evidence to best practice: effective implementation of change in patients' care. *Lancet* 362: 1225–1230.

Haas, M., Hall, J., Viney, R. et al. (2012). Breaking up is hard to do: why disinvestment in medical technology is harder than investment. *Australian Health Review* 36: 148–152.

Hailemariam, M., Bustos, T., Montgomery, B. et al. (2019). Evidence-based intervention sustainability strategies: a systematic review. *Implementation Science* 14: 57.

Heus, P., van Dulmen, S., Weenink, J. et al. (2023). What are effective strategies to reduce low-value care? an analysis of 121 randomized deimplementation studies. *Journal for Healthcare Quality* 10.1097.

Hofmann, B. (2021). Internal barriers to efficiency: why disinvestments are so difficult. Identifying and addressing internal barriers to disinvestment of health technologies. *Health Economics Policy and Law* 16: 473–488.

Laan, B.J., Maaskant, J.M., Spijkerman, I.J.B. et al. (2020). De-implementation strategy to reduce inappropriate use of intravenous and urinary catheters (RICAT): a multicentre, prospective, interrupted time-series and before and after study. *Lancet Infectious Diseases* 20: 864–872.

Lakhani, A., Lass, E., Silverstein, W.K. et al. (2016). Choosing wisely for medical education: six things medical students and trainees should question. *Academic Medicine* 91: 1374–1378.

Maher, L., Gustafson, D., and Evan, A. (2010). *Sustainability Model and Guide*. London: NHS Institute for innovation and improvement.

Parchman, M.L., Henrikson, N.B., Blasi, P.R. et al. (2017). Taking action on overuse: creating the culture for change. *Healthcare* 5: 199–203.

Parmelli, E., Flodgren, G., Beyer, F. et al. (2011). The effectiveness of strategies to change organisational culture to improve healthcare performance: a systematic review. *Implementation Science* 6: 33.

Pluye, P., Potvin, L., Denis, J.L. et al. (2004). Program sustainability: focus on organizational routines. *Health Promotion International* 19: 489–500.

Proctor, E., Luke, D., Calhoun, A. et al. (2015). Sustainability of evidence-based healthcare: research agenda, methodological advances, and infrastructure support. *Implementation Science* 10: 88.

Rosenbaum, L. and Lamas, D. (2012). Cents and sensitivity – teaching physicians to think about costs. *New England Journal of Medicine* 367: 99–101.

Scheirer, M.A., Hartling, G., and Hagerman, D. (2008). Defining sustainability outcomes of health programs: illustrations from an on-line survey. *Evaluation and Program Planning* 31: 335–346.

Shediac-Rizkallah, M.C. and Bone, L.R. (1998). Planning for the sustainability of community-based health programs: conceptual frameworks and future directions for research, practice and policy. *Health Education Research* 13: 87–108.

Shelton, R.C., Cooper, B.R., and Stirman, S.W. (2018). The sustainability of evidence-based interventions and practices in public health and health care. *Annual Review of Public Health* 39: 55–76.

Sorenson, C. and Japinga, M. (2022). Low-value care De-implementation: practices for systemwide reduction. *NEJM Catalyst Innovations in Care Delivery* 05: https://doi.org/10.1056/CAT.21.0387.

Van Egmond, S., Van Vliet, E.D., Wakkee, M. et al. (2022). Efficacy, cost-minimization, and budget impact of a personalized discharge letter for basal cell carcinoma patients to reduce low-value follow-up care. *PLoS One* 17: e0260978.

Vugt, S.V., De Schepper, E., Van Delft, S. et al. (2021). Effectiveness of professional and patient-oriented strategies in reducing vitamin D and B12 test ordering in primary care: a cluster randomised intervention study. *British Journal of General Practice Open* 5.

Wiltsey Stirman, S., Kimberly, J., Cook, N. et al. (2012). The sustainability of new programs and innovations: a review of the empirical literature and recommendations for future research. *Implementation Science* 7: 17.

# CHAPTER 12

# Training the Next Generation of Healthcare Providers to Address Overuse and Avoid Low-Value Care

Brian M. Wong[1], Christopher Moriates[2], Lorette Stammen[3], and Karen Born[4]

[1] Sunnybrook Health Sciences Centre, Centre for Quality Improvement and Patient Safety, University of Toronto, Toronto, Ontario, Canada
[2] Dell Medical School, University of Texas at Austin, Austin, Texas, USA
[3] School of Health Professions Education (SHE), Maastricht University, Maastricht, Limburg, The Netherlands
[4] Institute of Health Policy, Management & Evaluation, University of Toronto, Toronto, Ontario, Canada

*How to Reduce Overuse in Healthcare: A Practical Guide*, First Edition.
Edited by Tijn Kool, Andrea M. Patey, Simone van Dulmen, and Jeremy M. Grimshaw.
© 2024 John Wiley & Sons Ltd. Published 2024 by John Wiley & Sons Ltd.

## INTRODUCTION

This book primarily focusses on designing de-implementation interventions in clinical settings to reduce low-value care. But what if we could prevent low-value care from making it into clinical practice? Healthcare professionals' practice behaviours and patterns are the result of training experiences shaped by their clinical learning environment. Changing the way healthcare professionals are trained, focusing on the learning of high-value care, as well as supportive learning environments, may prevent the use of low-value care as learners progress through their careers. We present changes that are currently taking place and, in some instances, still need to take place in education and training to engage clinicians at their earliest stages of training to eliminate low-value care.

## HIGH-VALUE CARE COMPETENCIES

What abilities must health professionals demonstrate to contribute to high-value care practices in their clinical environment and thereby minimise the risk of providing low-value care? A critical first step to defining any educational change within a competency-based framework is to be clear about the desired outcomes of training. Training outcomes, often expressed as competencies, define those observable activities that learners must be able to demonstrate when they complete their training. Within the context of high-value care, commonly used frameworks, such as CanMEDS and the Accreditation Council for Graduate Medical Education Core Competencies (Frank et al. 2015), describe elements of high-value care in competencies such as health advocacy and systems-based practice. High-value, cost-conscious care (Weinberger 2011), value-based healthcare (Porter 2010), value-based medicine (Brown et al. 2005), reduction of low-value care, *Choosing Wisely* (Levinson et al. 2015), and the Institute for Healthcare Improvement Triple Aim (Berwick et al. 2008) are examples of concepts that have also drawn attention to high-value care. Although present in educational frameworks, it is important to acknowledge that attempts to structurally incorporate high-value education in undergraduate and postgraduate physician training have been met with variable success (Patel et al. 2014; Ryskina et al. 2018). This is partly due to the complexity of designing training that addresses high-value care by focusing on knowledge transmission, reflective practice, and a supportive environment (Stammen et al. 2015).

## TEACHING STUDENTS AND TRAINEES TO PROVIDE HIGH-VALUE CARE

A variety of approaches have supported students and trainees to learn about high-value care, ranging from formal teaching that transmits knowledge about high-value care concepts, including the reduction of healthcare interventions that do not provide benefits for patients (low-value care), to facilitation of reflective practice to give trainees insight into their past and current behaviour. However, such approaches must be bolstered by the creation of a supportive learning environment where the presence of positive faculty role models fosters a culture of high-value care that reinforces the desired training goals.

## EDUCATIONAL CHANGES TO THE FORMAL CURRICULUM

The formal curriculum is what we commonly think of when embarking on educational change: a lecture series, case rounds, online modules, or even a longitudinal project course. Changes to the formal curriculum represent important opportunities to introduce new concepts and principles to learners and develop the requisite knowledge, skills, and attitudes to deliver high-value care and reduce or eliminate low-value care. Formal education can be used to (i) increase knowledge; (ii) stimulate reflective practice; and (iii) create a supportive learning environment.

To increase knowledge, educational initiatives have focused on making learners aware of the cost of tests and treatments (in addition to general health economics principles), reviewing scientific evidence or published guidelines, and describing the various harms of low-value tests and treatments to both the patient and the health system (Stammen et al. 2015). Different teaching methods, such as lectures, small group learning, or pocket cards, have been used and demonstrated to have beneficial short-term impact on learning outcomes. Other examples include teaching learners about communication skills to counsel patients when requests arise for unnecessary tests or treatments (Mukerji et al. 2017). During these formal educational activities, faculty can help learners to reflect on behaviour and practice patterns through the use of prompts that can help to reinforce key concepts. Examples are: What unnecessary costs do patients bear when we order unnecessary tests and treatments? Why is it hard to counsel patients who are requesting an unnecessary test?

As mentioned earlier, attempts to integrate high-value care concepts into an already full curriculum can be challenging. Yet, for greatest impact on learning and culture change, concepts relating to high- and low-value care must be interwoven throughout the curriculum. We offer the following practical suggestions for ways to make changes to the formal curriculum to integrate high-value care principles.

First, it is critical to engage key stakeholders within the training programme, including educational leaders, faculty, and learners. Rather than simply emphasising the importance of high-value care as a new, stand-alone topic to highlight for learners in the training programme and advocating for time and space in the curriculum, we recommend linking high-value care content to training requirements that schools are already responsible for addressing. For example, the provision of high-value care could be framed within the context of promoting evidence-based practice including the avoidance of tests and treatments for which weak evidence exists, alongside advancing professionalism (Marcotte et al. 2020). It could also be framed as improving provider-patient communication and shared decision-making, or even larger curriculum redesign efforts such as the introduction of health system science as the 'third pillar' of medical education (Gonzalo et al. 2017).

Second, it is important to map the existing school's curriculum and identify opportunities to integrate high- and low-value care concepts into different lectures, case discussions, or other educational activities. Some schools organise their curriculum by organ system (e.g. cardiac, renal, etc.). So, for example, when students are learning approaches to the workup of chest pain during their cardiology instruction, concepts of trade-offs, costs, harms, and overuse should be incorporated into these lessons. A simple example from the University of Toronto in Canada was when students took the initiative to review the prior year's lecture slides and identified natural instances to incorporate *Choosing Wisely* recommendations and prepared a slide that they asked their professors to include during their lecture (Leon-Carlyle et al. 2015). Due to the physical and financial harms of low-value care, an emphasis may be placed on the physician responsibility to 'first, do not harm'.

Third, consider and leverage a broader range of learning experiences that training programmes use to integrate high-value care principles. Programmes that rely on case-based learning discussions could seek ways to make a subtopic for discussion related to high-value care and/or reducing low-value care. For example, case-based learning has been used to teach pharmacy students about relevant low-value care topics such as prescribing cascades and antimicrobial stewardship (Testman 2014; Nasr et al. 2022). A study involving German medical students demonstrated that the use of video can augment case-based learning about high-value care and improve short-term knowledge retention (Ludwig et al. 2018). Training on provider–patient communication can include role-play scenarios that feature patients seeking low-value interventions and helping learners to develop relevant skills related to empathy and shared decision-making (Mukerji et al. 2017).

Finally, many health professions training programmes now include health systems science and quality improvement (QI) as core training elements, often requiring learners to engage in a QI project. Programmes can list the reduction of low-value care practices as targets for learner-led initiatives, which both addresses important systems-based competencies related to high-value care and harnesses the power of learners to reduce unnecessary tests and treatments (Lam and Wong 2020).

## FACULTY ROLE MODELLING AND SUPPORTIVE LEARNING ENVIRONMENTS

Changes to the formal curriculum are necessary but rarely sufficient to drive change as much learning occurs through informal means. Informal learning is often unplanned and may even arise spontaneously in clinical settings. Discussions during case review in an ambulatory teaching clinic or ward rounds offer excellent opportunities for faculty to role-model high-value care practices and a focus on reducing low-value care.

The training environment imprints on learners and influences their future practice patterns. Residents who train in high-spending training environments become higher spending physicians, with the effect seen up to 15 years after graduation, even when the graduate moves and practices in a lower clinical care spending setting (Chen et al. 2014; Sirovich et al. 2014; Ryskina et al. 2015; Weng et al. 2020). Training environments that reinforce hierarchies and power imbalances between faculty and learners can impede open dialogue about low-value care practices and suppress learners who might want to 'speak up' when they observe low-value care practices and behaviours. Therefore, changing the culture and informal teaching within clinical learning environments can have far-reaching impacts on high-value care outcomes (see also Chapter 11).

To ingrain high-value care practices into daily clinical care delivery, programmes can introduce cognitive forcing functions, such as the Subjective, Objective, Assessment, Plan (SOAP-V) model that incorporates a 'Value' component within patient rounds presentations (Moser et al. 2016). The SOAP-V model prompts trainees when suggesting management plans to routinely ask themselves: (i) Will this change management? How does it incorporate evidence?; (ii) Have I considered the patient's goals?; (iii) What is the cost (actual or relative) of the test/treatment? The introduction of models such as SOAP-V can promote discussions between students, residents, and faculty related to reducing or avoiding routine areas of low-value care. Furthermore, these discussions can potentially create opportunities for learners to 'manage up' and share concepts that they have learned in the classroom regarding high-value care with faculty who likely did not have these concepts included during their formal medical education.

Making high-value care a shared goal for faculty and learners creates a supportive environment, opening up avenues for feedback on practices and critical discussions about obstacles to high-value care delivery. Faculty supervisors generally use three teaching methods to support high-value care delivery: Socratic questioning (more common in medical education), role modelling, and setting limits (Stammen et al. 2020). Supervisors can raise learners' awareness of high-value care-related issues through open-ended questions, such as those that are included in the SOAP-V model ('Will the result of that extra test change our treatment plan?'). They may also explore with the learner why they made a particular treatment decision, creating opportunities for shared reflection.

Faculty can intentionally role-model skills to help advance communication with patients about unnecessary testing or potentially inappropriate requests. In the presence of the learner, the faculty member may explain to a patient why a specific diagnostic intervention is not needed and discuss better alternatives. Supervising faculty can also intentionally role model by making their thinking visible, such as reasoning through a diagnostic decision with a learner, highlighting the pros and cons of a specific approach, and showing how they balance high-value care concepts. Lastly, supervisors could set limits on some practices, such as limiting learner autonomy where appropriate to prescribe specific expensive medications on their own

(Stammen et al. 2020). Setting limits needs to be balanced against local culture related to trainee autonomy and also appropriately adjusted as learners become more senior and are capable of making more independent decisions.

In addition to informal teaching, the 'hidden curriculum' is composed of unarticulated and often unintended lessons that can be powerful transmitters of norms, values, and beliefs that shape behaviours (Hafferty and Franks 1994). For example, learners may be congratulated for 'being thorough' or indirectly rewarded for suggesting rare diagnoses as part of a differential diagnosis, which might encourage ordering unnecessary, low-value tests. Educational conferences, such as morning reports, present an imbalanced focus on rare cases, rather than discussing common clinical scenarios, which reinforces expansive workups. Resident physicians are often asked by attending physicians about tests that were not ordered ('Why did not you get a chest x-ray this morning?') rather than questioning those that were ordered and may have been unnecessary (Moriates et al. 2013). To counteract these tendencies, faculty can instead purposefully 'celebrate restraint', such as highlighting when a trainee decides appropriately to NOT order a specific test or intervention (Detsky and Verma 2012). When hearing about a patient admitted overnight with syncope, the attending physician may say something like, 'Thank you for not ordering that head CT last night for this patient; you must have thought about it and you recognised that the patient did not need the head CT and was unlikely to benefit, so you appropriately avoided that test which is good for both the patient and the system'.

There is a role for trainees to help shape the informal and hidden curricula within clinical learning environments towards high-value care delivery and teaching. For example, a *Choosing Wisely* list for medical education was created with input provided from nearly 2000 medical students from across Canada (Lakhani et al. 2016). The list articulates six low-value practices that may occur in clinical learning environments which students and trainees should avoid (see Box 12.1).

## Box 12.1 Six Things Medical Students and Trainees Should Question

1. Do not suggest ordering the most invasive test or treatment before considering other less invasive option.
2. Do not suggest a test, treatment, or procedure that will not change the patient's clinical course.
3. Do not miss the opportunity to initiate conversations with patients about whether a test, treatment, or procedures is necessary.
4. Do not hesitate to ask for clarification on tests, treatments, or procedures that you believe are unnecessary.
5. Do not suggest ordering tests or performing procedures for the sole purpose of gaining personal clinical experience.
6. Do not suggest ordering tests or treatments preemptively for the sole purpose of anticipating what your supervisor would want.

*Source*: Adapted from Choosing Wisely Canada.

Students in other countries including in the Netherlands, New Zealand, and Japan have also created similar medical education lists citing low-value care practices to avoid. More recently, medical students at a handful of US medical schools recently created a 'Choosing Wisely Physician Excellence Award' to reinforce positive examples of faculty that support Choosing Wisely teaching and role modelling (Shields and Scott 2022). The students nominate faculty during their clinical rotations whose 'practice exemplifies high-value care' and the awardees publicly receive a lapel pin and certificate. Some schools, such as the University of Toronto, have even gone as far as creating annual awards for faculty and residents who demonstrate the virtues consistent with resource stewardship. In Japan, medical students crowdsourced cases and learner experiences to develop a handbook for trainees as a way to address the culture of high- and low-value care in medical education that they subsequently published and distributed widely (Soshi et al. 2017).

## ASSESSING HIGH-VALUE CARE LEARNING OUTCOMES

Assessment, the systematic collection and analysis of information to improve student learning by providing necessary feedback to support ongoing learning and growth, represents a critical element of a competency-based approach. Despite the rapid proliferation of literature supporting the teaching and learning of high-value care, there has been less published on approaches that support learner assessment. The following section provides an array of options for incorporating learner assessment into high-value care education.

One option involves leveraging existing assessment strategies and embedding high-value care elements. For example, Dell Medical School at The University of Texas at Austin incorporated criteria related to students' ability to apply concepts related to value. Examples are 'able to use value-based care i.e. considering patient preferences and costs when suggesting and justifying next steps', 'engages patient/family in shared decision-making', 'actively collaborates with other health professionals to coordinate care'. Other criteria are healthcare system context and leadership within clinical clerkship evaluations for all students across all rotations. One benefit of this approach is that it also messages to faculty and resident physicians completing these assessments the model of high-value care delivery that the institution is aiming to achieve, purposefully contributing to the hidden curriculum of what is celebrated locally.

We see examples of this approach emerging more explicitly within national training standards. In Canada, as part of the implementation of competency-based education for specialist training, each specialty has defined a list of entrustable professional activities (EPAs), which are the key tasks of their discipline that are made up of several sub-competencies. For example, an EPA for internal medicine training is to 'assess, diagnose, and manage patients with complex acute medical presentations'. One of the competencies specifically mentions the importance of 'demonstrating resource stewardship in clinical care'. These assessment approaches draw from CanMEDS, a physician competency framework that has been taken up by approximately 50 countries internationally (Frank et al. 2015).

There are also examples of assessment tools specifically designed to assess high-value care competencies (Alliance for Academic Internal Medicine 2022). For instance, an important high-value care competency relates to effective communication with patients and families when addressing requests for unnecessary tests and treatments. A structured assessment tool exists that uses a rating scale to assess residents' ability to provide clear recommendations, elicit patient concerns, demonstrate empathy, and arrive at a shared decision. Such a tool could be used in a variety of different settings, ranging from the clinical workplace to simulated assessment such as an objective structured clinical exam. Similarly, tools have been created to support the assessment of QI projects, which programmes commonly use to engage learners in system change initiatives aimed at improving high-value care.

## ENABLERS OF EDUCATIONAL CHANGE

Like with any new topic in health professions education, change can be leveraged through a number of different mechanisms. These include revisions to competency frameworks, addition of new questions to certification exams and changes to training standards, and accreditation to name a few. Such changes are already starting to occur; many physician competency frameworks now explicitly list high-value care competencies, and certification exams, such as the American Board of Internal Medicine exam, include questions where the correct answer is to demonstrate appropriate conservative management and *not* order the test. The National Board of Medical Examiners in the US has introduced a Health Systems Science Examination as a standardised assessment for medical students, with high-value care comprising approximately a quarter of the questions. The inclusion of a Health Systems Science 'shelf exam' within undergraduate medical education raises the importance and perceived relevance of this topic for many students, as no longer is learning components of high-value care something that is 'not on the test' and, thus, may be seen as extraneous.

An important global driver of change within medical training resulted from the Students and Trainees Advocating for Resource Stewardship (STARS) programme. STARS was first established by the *Choosing Wisely Canada* campaign in 2015 (Cardone et al. 2017). The goal of STARS was to seed a medical student-led, grassroots movement in support of increased awareness of resource stewardship in medical education. STARS engaged two medical student leaders from each of Canada's 17 medical schools on an annual basis, and these students led local initiatives in support of resource stewardship including developing student interest groups, hosting conferences, journal clubs, and working with faculty to embed resource stewardship content into the curriculum. The programme is flexible and intended to enable student leadership to advance resource stewardship addressing local needs and contexts. Since STARS launched in 2015, the programme model has spread to seven countries with active STARS or student-led campaigns in support of national *Choosing Wisely* campaigns in the US, the Netherlands, Italy, Japan, Brazil, Norway, and New Zealand (Born et al. 2019). There are shared attributes of the model across multiple countries, which include that students who are involved have the opportunity to advance knowledge in resource stewardship in medicine specifically through enhanced content and presentations from experts on the topic.

## ALIGNING CONTINUING PROFESSIONAL DEVELOPMENT AND QUALITY IMPROVEMENT

While much of this chapter focuses attention on students and trainees, we would be remiss if we did not acknowledge that clinicians in practice must also demonstrate competencies necessary to deliver high-value care even if they did not acquire them during their training. This challenge exists for many emerging topics, such that educational change efforts that seek to advance high-value care practices amongst clinicians must include a continuing professional development (CPD) component.

While beyond the scope of this chapter, we acknowledge that the field of CPD is undergoing evolution with a shift away from traditional forms of CPD that tend to be more passive and focus primarily on knowledge transfer such as lecture presentations and conferences. Educational approaches known to promote high-value care and reduce low-value practices such as reflective practice and simulated communication training mentioned earlier are consistent with contemporary CPD practices and are relevant for clinicians in practice as well. There is also a growing recognition that CPD should target behaviour and practice change and requires more active forms of learning that emphasise interprofessionalism, workplace-based activities, and, most importantly, QI (Shojania et al. 2012).

This shift is occurring amidst calls for greater alignment between CPD and QI, given that both CPD and QI ultimately share the same goal of improved patient outcomes. Interestingly, in some jurisdictions, we are now seeing both regulatory and certifying bodies enact requirements for active involvement in QI activities as part of ongoing licensure and maintenance of certification. This alignment of incentives may serve as an important driver towards clinician engagement in practice-based de-- implementation activities.

## KEY POINTS

- Health professional education must start upstream and introduce high-value care concepts early in training to develop the necessary skills to avoid low-value tests and treatments.
- Attention must be paid to formal curriculum to ensure the transmission of knowledge related to high-value care practices, while also fostering informal learning opportunities

through reflective practice and faculty role modelling (see Table 12.1 for a summary of key approaches).

- Curriculum change requires the engagement of key educational stakeholders, curriculum mapping, and leveraging of existing learning activities to integrate high- and low-value care concepts into different lectures, case discussions, or other educational activities
- Enablers of educational change should combine top-down and bottom-up approaches to increase learner awareness about the dangers of low-value care practices and promote high-value care culture such as the STARS student-led movement.

**TABLE 12.1** Examples for incorporating high-value care principles into formal and informal learning in health professions education.

| Educational approach | Illustrative example |
|---|---|
| *Formal curriculum* | |
| Align high-value care concepts to content areas already required in training | Frame provision of high-value care in the context of evidence-based medicine, professionalism, patient-provide communication, or health-systems science. |
| Add Choosing Wisely campaign recommendations to existing lectures and case discussions | During 'cardiology' week, include a reference to Choosing Wisely recommendations that highlight low-value cardiac tests and treatments to avoid |
| Leverage case-based learning to incorporate discussions about high and low-value care | Case-based seminars for pharmacy students could include topics such as the harms of prescribing cascades or antimicrobial stewardship |

**TABLE 12.1** (Continued)

| Educational approach | Illustrative example |
|---|---|
| Move beyond knowledge transfer to develop necessary skills to reduce low-value care | Use simulation to students how to counsel patients and engage in effective shared decision-making to address requests for low-value tests and treatments |
| Engage learners in quality improvement initiatives aimed at reducing low-value care | Programmes that have a quality improvement project requirement can list the reduction of low-value care practices as a target for learner-led improvement initiatives |
| *Informal curriculum* | |
| Introduce cognitive forcing functions | The SOAP-V model incorporates a 'value' component within patient round presentations to prompt students to consider how their management plans address low-value care |
| Socratic questioning | Faculty can ask open-ended questions such as 'will the results of this test change our management plan?' to generate discussion and reflection |
| Intentional role modelling by faculty | Intentional faculty role-modelling behaviours include making their thinking and diagnostic reasoning visible to highlight the pros and cons of a particular diagnostic approach |
| Providing feedback and setting limits | Faculty can provide feedback to help correct low-value practices and set limits where appropriate, making sure to achieve a balance between clinical supervision and learning autonomy |
| Celebrating restraint | When learners choose not to order low-value tests and/or treatments, faculty can make specific mention of this and provide positive reinforcement |

## SOURCES

Faculty may share *Choosing Wisely* lists or other resources such as articles from *JAMA Internal Medicine's* 'Less is More' series (https://jamanetwork.com/collections/44045/less-is-more) or *Journal of Hospital Medicine's* 'Things We Do For No Reason' series (https://shmpublications.onlinelibrary.wiley.com/index/15535606?startPage=&ContentItem Category=CHOOSING%20WISELY®%3A%20THINGS %20WE%20DO%20FOR%20NO%20REASON) with their clinical teams to generate discussion regarding common areas of overuse within their field, inviting reflection about local practices.

## REFERENCES

Alliance for Academic Internal Medicine. (2022). High-Value Care Learner Assessment Tools. https://www.im.org/resources/ume-gme--program-resources/hvc/hvc-assessment (accessed August 19 2022).

Berwick, D.M., Nolan, T.W., and Whittington, J. (2008). The triple aim: care, health, and cost. *Health Affairs* 27: 759–769.

Born, K.B., Moriates, C., Valencia, V. et al. (2019). Learners as leaders: a global groundswell of students leading choosing wisely initiatives in medical education. *Academic Medicine* 94: 1699–1703.

Brown, M.M., Brown, G.C., and Sharma, S. (2005). *Evidence-Based to Value-Based Medicine*. Chicago: American Medical Association.

Cardone, F., Cheung, D., Han, A. et al. (2017). Choosing Wisely Canada students and trainees advocating for resource stewardship (STARS) campaign: a descriptive evaluation. *Canadian Medical Association Open Access Journal* 5: E864–E871.

Chen, C., Petterson, S., Phillips, R. et al. (2014). Spending patterns in region of residency training and subsequent expenditures for care provided by practicing physicians for Medicare beneficiaries. *Journal of American Medical Association* 312: 2385–2393.

Detsky, A.S. and Verma, A.A. (2012). A new model for medical education: celebrating restraint. *Joournal of the American Medical Association* 308: 1329–1330.

Frank, J.R., Snell, L., Sherbino, J., et al. (2015). CanMEDS 2015 Physician Competency Framework Canada, R.C.O.P.a.S.O.

Gonzalo, J.D., Haidet, P., Papp, K.K. et al. (2017). Educating for the 21st-century health care system: an interdependent framework of basic, clinical, and systems sciences. *Academic Medicine* 92: 35–39.

Hafferty, F.W. and Franks, R. (1994). The hidden curriculum, ethics teaching, and the structure of medical education. *Academic Medicine* 69: 861–871.

Lakhani, A., Lass, E., Silverstein, W.K. et al. (2016). Choosing Wisely for medical education: six things medical students and trainees should question. *Academic Medicine* 91: 1374–1378.

Lam, P.W. and Wong, B.M. (2020). Harnessing the power of residents as change agents in quality improvement. *Academic Medicine* 96: 21–23.

Leon-Carlyle, M., Srivastava, R., and Levinson, W. (2015). Choosing Wisely Canada: integrating stewardship in medical education. *Academic Medicine: Journal of the Association of American Medical Colleges* 90: 1430.

Levinson, W., Kallewaard, M., Bhatia, R.S. et al. (2015). 'Choosing Wisely': a growing international campaign. *BMJ Quality and Safety* 24: 167–174.

Ludwig, S., Schuelper, N., Brown, J. et al. (2018). How can we teach medical students to choose wisely? A randomised controlled cross-over study of video-versus text-based case scenarios. *BMC Medicine* 16: 1–9.

Marcotte, L.M., Moriates, C., Wolfson, D.B. et al. (2020). Professionalism as the bedrock of high-value care. *Academic Medicine* 95: 864–867.

Moriates, C., Shah, N., and Arora, V.M. (2013). Medical training and expensive care. *Health Affairs* 32: 196.

Moser, E.M., Huang, G.C., Packer, C.D. et al. (2016). SOAP-V: introducing a method to empower medical students to be change agents in bending the cost curve. *Journal of Hospital Medicine* 11: 217–220.

Mukerji, G., Weinerman, A., Schwartz, S. et al. (2017). Communicating wisely: teaching residents to communicate effectively with patients and caregivers about unnecessary tests. *BMC Medical Education* 17: 1–6.

Nasr, Z.G., Moustafa, D.A.H., Dahmani, S. et al. (2022). Investigating pharmacy students' therapeutic decision-making with respect to anti-microbial stewardship cases. *BMC Medical Education* 22: 1–8.

Patel, M.S., Reed, D.A., Loertscher, L. et al. (2014). Teaching residents to provide cost-conscious care: a national survey of residency program directors. *JAMA Internal Medicine* 174: 470–472.

Porter, M.E. (2010). What is value in health care? *New England Journal of Medicine* 363: 2477–2481.

Ryskina, K.L., Halpern, S.D., Minyanou, N.S. et al. (2015). The role of training environment care intensity in US physician cost consciousness. In: *Mayo Clinic Proceedings*, 313–320. Elsevier.

Ryskina, K.L., Holmboe, E.S., Shea, J.A. et al. (2018). Physician experiences with high value care in internal medicine residency: mixed-methods study of 2003–2013 residency graduates. *Teaching and Learning in Medicine* 30: 57–66.

Shields, C.A. and Scott, R.E. (2022). Student-nominated awards recognizing Attendings' desirable behaviors. *Academic Medicine* http://dx.doi.org/10.1097/ACM.0000000000004384.

Shojania, K.G., Silver, I., and Levinson, W. (2012). Continuing medical education and quality improvement: a match made in heaven? *Annals of Internal Medicine* 156: 305–308.

Sirovich, B.E., Lipner, R.S., Johnston, M. et al. (2014). The association between residency training and internists' ability to practice conservatively. *JAMA Internal Medicine* 174: 1640–1648.

Soshi, M., Maeda, K., Isoda, S. et al. (2017). Dawn of Choosing Wisely Japan student committee. *Journal of General and Family Medicine* 18: 487.

Stammen, L.A., Stalmeijer, R.E., Paternotte, E. et al. (2015). Training physicians to provide high-value, cost-conscious care: a systematic review. *Journal of the American Medical Association* 314: 2384–2400.

Stammen, L.A., Driessen, E.W., Notermans, C.C. et al. (2020). How do attending physicians prepare residents to deliver high-value, cost-conscious care? *Academic Medicine* 95: 764.

Testman, J.A. (2014). The prescribing cascade game: applying geriatric pharmacotherapy principles in the classroom. *Currents in Pharmacy Teaching and Learning* 6: 646–651.

Weinberger, S.E. (2011). Providing high-value, cost-conscious care: a critical seventh general competency for physicians. *Annals of Internal Medicine* 155: 386–388.

Weng, W., Van Parys, J., Lipner, R.S. et al. (2020). Association of regional practice environment intensity and the ability of internists to practice high-value care after residency. *JAMA Network Open* 3: e202494–e202494.

# CHAPTER 13

# Examples from Clinical Practice

Simone van Dulmen[1], Daniëlle Kroon[1], Tijn Kool[1], Kyle Kirkham[2], and Johanna Caro Mendivelso[3,4]

[1] Department of IQ Healthcare, Radboud University Medical Center, Radboud Institute for Health Sciences, Nijmegen, The Netherlands
[2] Department of Anaesthesia and Pain Management, Toronto Western Hospital, University of Toronto, Toronto, Canada
[3] CIBER de Epidemiología y Salud Pública (CIBERESP), Madrid, Spain
[4] Agency for Health Quality and Assessment of Catalonia, Barcelona, Spain

## INTRODUCTION

In the scientific literature, many studies report on the specific phases in the de-implementation process. For example, there are studies reporting on the volume of low-value care (Muskens et al. 2021), describing frameworks (Walsh-Bailey et al. 2021), identification of barriers and facilitators (van Dulmen et al. 2020; Augustsson et al. 2021), studies on methodology (Upvall and Bourgault 2018; Prusaczyk et al. 2020), effectiveness of

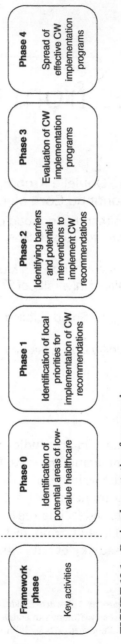

**FIGURE 13.1** De-implementation framework.

interventions (Niven et al. 2015), and a limited studies reporting on long-term effects and spread of the results (Clyne et al. 2016). Only a few studies report on all the different phases of the de-implementation project, but they are rarely reporting on all the phases in one article (Almazan et al. 2022).

This chapter is filling this gap by providing examples of de-implementation projects following the steps of the framework as described in Chapter 4 (see Figure 13.1), aiming to guide the reader with a clear picture of the types of interventions, influencing factors, and outcome measures. This supports the reader to make a translation to situations in their own practice. We illustrate the process by describing the identified problem, choosing the strategy, the way it is delivered, monitored, and evaluated, and how it was disseminated.

The examples provided will be from different countries, health systems, type of stakeholder, and strategies. The examples are so diverse that together they offer a wide spectrum to learn from. We limit ourselves to examples, because otherwise a very large list of possible (combinations of) interventions would arise. It is impossible to be complete as the number of possible interventions is enormous, and this must be specifically linked to the influencing factors for the specific situation. We will provide additional information on what can be learned from this example.

**Example 1: Reduce overuse of laboratory testing in clinical setting, the Netherlands.**

| Phase | |
|---|---|
| 0. Identification of low value areas | Inappropriate use of laboratory tests is a well-recognised phenomenon, and overuse rates of approximately 20% have been reported (Zhi et al. 2013). |
| | Appropriate laboratory testing is also one of the Choosing Wisely recommendations of the Dutch Association of Internal Medicine. |
| 1. Identification of local priorities for implementation | Diagnostic laboratory testing in the internal medicine department (inpatient, outpatient, and emergency medicine) of four teaching hospitals. |
| 2. Identifying barriers and interventions | Barriers/facilitators were identified by questionnaires during the pre-intervention period and during the intervention period. Questionnaire 'Willingness to change', categorised in Model 'Grol and Wensing': individual factors, social factors, organisational factors, and environmental factors (Grol et al. 2013). |
| | The most important barriers were difficulties in data retrieval, difficulties with incorporation of new working agreements in daily practice, and high resident turnover. The most important facilitators were education, continuous attention for overuse of diagnostic testing, feedback, residents' involvement, and involvement of local champions (experienced clinical role models) (Bindraban et al. 2019) |
| | The interventions performed in this project were partly derived from previous literature in which the interventions aimed at changing behaviour and attitude were divided into the following categories: education, audit and feedback methods, (computerised) provider order entry system changes, and others. |

All participating hospitals were given the opportunity to focus on the specific facets of the intervention as deemed useful and possible in the local situation, thus 'tailoring' their interventions.

The main interventions that the hospitals choose were intensified supervision, creating awareness, and modifications in (computerised) order entry systems. Intensified supervision of residents by senior physicians refers to explicitly focusing on indications for ordering laboratory tests and asking critical questions ('Does the result of this test add value for diagnostics, treatment, or prognosis?', 'Is repetition of this test necessary at this moment?', 'Is it necessary to order these tests combined?') during morning reports, daily supervision meetings, grand rounds, and other clinical meetings.

3. Evaluation

A multi-centre before–after study was conducted at the internal medicine departments (inpatient, outpatient, and emergency departments) of four hospitals in the Netherlands.

4. Spread and preserve effect

The primary outcome measure was the diagnostic laboratory test order volume in the internal medicine department (inpatient, outpatient, and emergency department).

Secondary outcomes were laboratory expenditure, order volumes and expenditure for other diagnostic modalities, and clinical patient outcomes.

(Continued)

(Continued)

**Phase**

Laboratory test volume per patient contact decreased by 11.4% in the four hospitals, whereas the volume increased by 2.4% in 19 comparable hospitals without an intervention. Clinical outcomes were not associated with negative changes.

A questionnaire was used to evaluate the process and which factors were of greatest influence, categorised in Model 'Grol and Wensing': individual factors, social factors, organisational factors, environmental factors.

Important facilitators in the project were education, continuous attention for diagnostic testing, and feedback. Involvement of clinical chemists and establishing clear working agreements were also considered important. During the project, the teams were expanded with physicians representing internal medicine subspecialties. This facilitated the gain of widespread support, which was a crucial element in the project. Having enthusiastic internists and residents function as role models was considered a strong facilitator. Members of the coordinating project team considered the involvement of residents as the main factor contributing to the success of the project.

The most important barrier was obtaining reliable real-time data on ordering volumes and costs, which made it difficult to monitor progress in some clinics. In addition, it took several months before reduction efforts translated into consistent changes in ordering patterns. Although modifying the order systems was an important facilitator, yet their rigidness was seen as a barrier in one hospital (Bindraban et al. 2019).

Spreading: In a national project the interventions were spread to other hospitals in the Netherlands. A scaling team informed the interested hospitals about the intervention and presented in a meeting with the local team concrete do's and don'ts and provided personalized advise. This enabled the local teams to select the targeted intervention components tailored to the local context. The scaling team was approachable for all questions during the conduction of the intervention. In addition, The scaling team organised meetings with the learning community, including all local teams. During these meetings, the hospitals shared data, discussed difficulties and successes.

Preserving results: A follow-up study showed that laboratory volume reductions have significantly sustained in both hospitals over 22 months. One hospita flattened the number of laboratory test in the follow-up period, whereas in the other hospital the testing volume steadily increased towards the pre-intervention level. The awareness about appropriate testing was maintained, and facets that were compatible with the daily practice and automated were better preserved than facets that lacked profit or required a substantial time investment.

A sustainable reduction is possible; contextual factors differed between hospitals, so targeted interventions to sustain the reduction are necessary. After the ending of the study period, sustained attention and awareness is needed in order to preserve the results.

Contributors

Renuka Bindraban, Prabath W.B. Nanayakkara, Marlou van Beneden, Roos Boerman, Daniëlle Kroon

**Example 2: Essencial Initiative, Spain.**

| Phase | Essencial Initiative |
|---|---|
| 0. Identification of low value areas | The Essencial Initiative is a public policy project from the Catalan Agency for Healthcare Quality and Assessment of Catalonia (AQuAS) that aims to identify low-value clinical practices, and to elaborate recommendations to avoid them (Essencial 2022a). It started in 2013, and in 2015, the de-implementation process gradually began in 169 primary care teams (PCTs) in eight different pilots in Catalonia. A PCT is a multidisciplinary team providing primary care services including family physicians, nurses, paediatricians, social workers, dentists, among others. |
| | According to their preferences, each PCT chose which Essencial recommendations to work on. The top five selected were: (i) Proton-pump inhibitors in patients over 65 years or with polypharmacy, (ii) Statins in population with low or moderate coronary risk, (iii) PSA screening, (iv) Bisphosphonates in postmenopausal women with low risk of fractures, and (v) Benzodiazepines for insomnia in elderly patients (Almazan et al. 2022). In this example experience, we present one pilot with 11 PCT from different regions in Catalonia and the results of one recommendation: Statins in population with low or moderate coronary risk. |
| 1. Identification of local priorities for implementation | The recommendation to avoid Statins in population with low coronary risk was elaborated in the Essencial Initiative (evidence based medicine recommendations): 'Systematic prescription of statins for primary prevention cardiovascular disease is not recommended in patients who present low coronary risk' (Essencial 2022b). |

| | |
|---|---|
| 2. Identifying barriers and interventions | A qualitative approach was used to identify barriers and solutions through a focus group within each PCT formed by clinical leaders, who would act as local champions for the promotion of the project.

Professionals generally identified five groups of barriers: (i) practitioners' behaviour (such as lack of knowledge, disagreement among team members or clinical inertia), (ii) physician–patient relationship (mainly confidence and trust), (iii) lack of integrated pathways between hospital and primary care settings (proximity between PCT and hospital, care continuity of processes or alliances), (iv) industry pressure, and (v) external factors (e.g. insufficient visiting time) and lack of resources (equipment).

Specifically for the statins recommendation, identified barriers included: (i) a culture of excessive and early medicalisation, without promoting healthy lifestyle habits, (ii) allowing time for behavioural changes to consolidate, (iii) lack of culture in preventive medical visits, (iv) patient's preference for medication rather than changing lifestyle, (v) lack of awareness of side effects, and (vi) not estimating through validated tools the cardiovascular risk.

The leader with the PCT elaborated a Plan of Action which included a selection of the recommendations to be implemented by the team, identified barriers of the low-value clinical practices and proposals of interventions to deal with these drivers.

In a focus group four themes of solutions were identified to overcome the barriers: (i) patient empowerment (e.g. promote awareness of their health), (ii) training for professionals (mainly providing tools for decision making, communication skills), (iii) organisational change, and (iv) integrated pathways between primary care setting and others healthcare settings. |

(Continued)

(Continued)

| Phase | Essencial Initiative |
|---|---|
| | The team developed monitoring indicators to assess the progress related to each recommendation. A monthly follow-up of the indicators was provided to each participating PCT using a real world data visualisation tool. For each of the low-value practice identified, baseline indicators were provided to the clinical teams and monitored throughout the project. |
| | Feedback was provided as an intervention in all PCTs. Other interventions specifics to statins included: (i) Informative and formative meeting with the team, (ii) external communication: leaflets, information on local media, (iii) promoting ongoing training, (iv) standardise the information and scales to be used at consultation, and (vi) integrated pathways between primary care and hospitals. |
| 3. Evaluation | An uncontrolled before–after study was implemented. Eleven PCT from different regions in Catalonia participated in the pilot project throughout 24 months. The primary outcome measure was the prevalence of statins in population with low or moderate cardiovascular risk. Secondary outcomes were clinician knowledge and perceptions of the recommendation. |
| | The PCTs that selected the recommendation to avoid statins in population with low or moderate coronary risk had a decline in the percentage of inadequacy from 13.2% at baseline to 8.3% after 24 months, which accounts for a 37.0% reduction. |
| | Nevertheless, it is not possible to attribute these results only to this project, because there are more initiatives at primary care level aligned with Essencial in terms of reducing overdiagnosis and overtreatment. |

Brainstorming and open questionnaires were carried out to evaluate the process. The initiative was generally well received, but some professionals thought that the project was aimed to 'budget cuts' (ow-value clinical practices were relatec to waste, cost-opportunity). It was necessary to modulate the message and tc stress that the objective was to foster quality of healthcare and improve patient's safety.

The facilitators included the participation in the de-implementation of low-value clinical practices was voluntary, and the recommendations for de-implementation were identified by professionals at the local level. The quality indicator information system allowed to share and monitor information at individual and team levels.

Spread: The indicators with real world data created for the follow-up of the de-implementation project were later available in all of the Catalan territory. As a consequence, other PCTs and some hospitals spontaneously started to implement Essencial recommendations. Additionally, the indicators are still nowadays available, so PCT can continue monitoring their performance related to these low-value clinical practices.

Preserve the results: In Catalonia, the inadequacy of the treatment with statins was estimated in 2015 in 8.4% and in 2C21 was 5.1%. After the pilots have ended, we have continued to observe a decrease towards safer statin prescription patterns.

4. Spread and preserve effect

(Continued)

| Phase | Essencial Initiative |
|---|---|
| | The Essencial Initiative's role is to transfer knowledge about low-value clinical practices and advocate for a cultural change towards high-value care, as well as to help with the monitoring through the design of indicators. Lessons learned about the Essencial Initiative are: |
| | – As healthcare professionals are key leaders in the change of clinical practices, a bottom-up strategy should be encouraged. Nonetheless, they need support from the organisations for change to happen, and therefore, managers should also be committed too. |
| | – In our experience, all element interventions to de-implement low-value care practice were similar, but the way they are delivered were different between the organisations. However, it would be advisable to standardise interventions, in order to generate solid evidence on implementation science so that successful interventions can be scaled up. |
| | – Alignment between two levels of attention unifying protocols and standard procedures and recommendations is necessary to overcome the lack of integrated pathways between hospital and primary care setting. |
| | – Cultural change takes time, and the participation of key actors (healthcare professionals and patients) in the project, alongside other stakeholders, is crucial to promote the change. |
| | – There is a need of involvement from healthcare professionals, patients, and citizens in communication strategies to find a better way to adapt the message to the main stakeholders. |
| Contributors | Johanna Caro Mendivelso, Cari Almazán Saez, Garazi Carrillo Aguirre, Helena Bentué Jiménez |

**Example 3: Reducing unnecessary preoperative tests for patients having low-risk surgeries – the ESPRESS study, Canada.**

| Phase | |
|---|---|
| 0. Identification of low value areas | The Canadian Anaesthesiologists' Society established its Top five Choosing Wisely Canada recommendations, which focus on low-value tests in ambulatory surgery. They recommend that investigations should not be ordered on a routine basis, but should be based on the patient's health status, drug therapy, and with consideration to the proposed surgical intervention. |
| | Many preoperative tests (e.g. electrographs and chest X-rays) are routinely ordered for, and the subsequent test results are rarely used. In addition, unnecessary testing may lead physicians to pursue and treat borderline and false-positive laboratory abnormalities. |
| 1. Identification of local priorities for implementation | Administrative data from the Institute of Clinical Evaluative Sciences (ICES), demonstrated overuse of low-value tests and a significant inter-hospital variation across 137 Ontario hospitals (Kirkham et al. 2015). Thirty one percent of all patients received an electrocardiograph (ECG) but the rate of this test showed a 26-fold variation across hospitals in the Canadian province of Ontario. |
| | Key Ontario health system leaders met to identify Choosing Wisely Ontario priorities for implementation and a key initial hospital priority was preoperative testing prior to ambulatory surgery. |

(Continued)

(Continued)

| Phase | |
|---|---|
| 2. Identifying barriers and interventions | Theoretical Domains Framework (TDF; see Chapter 8) was used to interview Ontario anaesthesiologists and surgeons to identify key factors that participants believed contributed to overuse of preoperative tests (Patey et al. 2012).

Findings included conflicting comments about who was responsible for the test ordering (TDF domain – Social/professional role and identity), inability to cancel tests ordered by fellow physicians (Beliefs about capabilities and Social influences), and the problem with tests being completed before the anaesthesiologists see the patient (Beliefs about capabilities and Environmental context and resources). There were also concerns that not testing might be associated with harms (overnight admissions, re-admissions).

Findings from the study described above led to the development of a multicomponent intervention, which focused on increasing accountability in the healthcare system for preoperative test ordering.

The intervention consisted of (i) Changing hospital policy to prevent test ordering, (ii) Identifying a local champion to support hospital policy change, (iii) Delivering an education workshop to inform and support teams of policy change, and (iv) Restructuring of patient flow and responsibility to prevent unnecessary tests. |
| 3. Evaluation | Interrupted time series in nine-year historic and 12 months post-intervention. This approach provided a total of 36 pre-intervention intervals (quarterly for nine years). Post-intervention, data were collected for 24 months, similarly divided into quarterly intervals.

Outcome measure included the number of preoperative investigations conducted per patient. This will also be compared between the intervention and control sites. |

Our study in one hospital of the proposed intervention led to a 48% reduction in low-value preoperative ECGs.

No process evaluation or economic evaluation was conducted for this study.

| | |
|---|---|
| 4. Spread and preserve effect | We are currently conducting a parallel two-arm cluster randomised control trial with repeated cross-sectional measurements before and after intervention in 22 Ontario hospitals. Recruitment of hospitals has started in January of 2023.

Outcome measure included the number of preoperative investigations conducted per patient will also be compared between the intervention and control sites. Additionally, individual rates of same-day surgery cancellation, overnight admission, re-operation in 24 hours, return visits to health care provider within 7 days were measured as well as 30-day all-cause mortality from the date of surgery.

Alongside the trial, we plan to include a process evaluation to determine whether the intervention is delivered as designed (fidelity); to determine whether any changes in low-value preoperative test ordering are mediated through changes to the perceived barriers/enablers (mechanism of action); and to understand partici-pants' experiences of the intervention.

Economic impact of the policy change will be examined through the following outcomes:

1. Total preoperative investigation cost within 30 days pre-surgery, before and after the WCH policy change for each site, and between the intervention and control sites; |

(Continued)

(Continued)

| Phase | |
|---|---|
| | 2. Total health care costs within 7 days post-surgery before and after the WCH policy change for each site, and between the intervention and control sites; |
| | 3. Total health care costs 30 days within post-surgery before and after the WCH policy change for each site, and between the intervention and control sites. |
| | If we determine the intervention is effective, it could be rolled out across Ontario to reduce these low-value tests. |
| Contributors | Kyle Kirkham, Richard Brull, Muhammad Mamdani, Isaranuwatchai Wanrudee, Danielle Martin |

# REFERENCES

Almazan, C., Caro-Mendivelso, J.M., Mias, M. et al. (2022). Catalan experience of deadoption of low-value practices in primary care. *BMJ Quality and Safety* 11: e001065.

Augustsson, H., Ingvarsson, S., Nilsen, P. et al. (2021). Determinants for the use and de-implementation of low-value care in health care: a scoping review. *Implementation Science Communication* 2: 13.

Bindraban, R.S., Van Beneden, M., Kramer, M.H.H. et al. (2019). Association of a Multifaceted Intervention with Ordering of unnecessary laboratory tests among caregivers in internal medicine departments. *JAMA Network Open* 2: e197577.

Clyne, B., Smith, S.M., Hughes, C.M. et al. (2016). Sustained effectiveness of a multifaceted intervention to reduce potentially inappropriate prescribing in older patients in primary care (OPTI-SCRIPT study). *Implementation Science* 11: 79.

Essencial. (2022a). Essencial Salut. Essencial Initiative. https://essencialsalut.gencat.cat/en/inici (accessed 9 Apirl 2022).

Essencial. (2022b). Statins in population with low or moderate coronary risk. Essencial Initiative. https://essencialsalut.gencat.cat/en/detalls/Article/estatines_risc_coronari (accessed 9 Apirl 2022).

Grol, R., Wensing, M., Eccles, M.P. et al. (2013). *Improving Patient Care: The Implementation of Change in Health Care*. Wiley.

Kirkham, K.R., Wijeysundera, D.N., Pendrith, C. et al. (2015). Preoperative testing before low-risk surgical procedures. *Canadian Medical Association Journal* 187: E349–E358.

Muskens, J., Kool, R.B., Van Dulmen, S.A. et al. (2021). Overuse of diagnostic testing in healthcare: a systematic review. *BMJ Quality and Safety* https://doi.org/10.1136/bmjqs-2020-012576.

Niven, D.J., Mrklas, K.J., Holodinsky, J.K. et al. (2015). Towards understanding the de-adoption of low-value clinical practices: a scoping review. *BMC Medicine* 13: 255.

Patey, A.M., Islam, R., Francis, J.J. et al. (2012). Anesthesiologists' and surgeons' perceptions about routine pre-operative testing in low-risk patients: application of the theoretical domains framework (TDF) to identify factors that influence physicians' decisions to order pre-operative tests. *Implementation Science* 7: 52.

Prusaczyk, B., Swindle, T., and Curran, G. (2020). Defining and conceptualizing outcomes for de-implementation: key distinctions from implementation outcomes. *Implementation Science Communication* 1: 43.

Upvall, M.J. and Bourgault, A.M. (2018). De-implementation: a concept analysis. *Nursing Forum* http://dx.doi.org/10.1111/nuf.12256.

Van Dulmen, S.A., Naaktgeboren, C.A., Heus, P. et al. (2020). Barriers and facilitators to reduce low-value care: a qualitative evidence synthesis. *BMJ Open* 10: e040025.

Walsh-Bailey, C., Tsai, E., Tabak, R.G. et al. (2021). A scoping review of de-implementation frameworks and models. *Implementation Science* 16: 100.

Zhi, M., Ding, E.L., Theisen-Toupal, J. et al. (2013). The landscape of inappropriate laboratory testing: a 15-year meta-analysis. *PLoS One* 8: e78962.

# CHAPTER 14

# Starting Tomorrow

Tijn Kool[1], Andrea M. Patey[2,3], Jeremy M. Grimshaw[2,3,4], and Simone van Dulmen[1]

[1] Department of IQ Healthcare, Radboud University Medical Center, Radboud Institute for Health Sciences, Nijmegen, The Netherlands
[2] Centre for Implementation Research, Ottawa Hospital Research Institute, Ottawa, Ontario, Canada
[3] School of Epidemiology and Public Health, University of Ottawa, Ottawa, Ontario, Canada
[4] Department of Medicine, University of Ottawa, Ottawa, Ontario, Canada

Medical overuse is a serious problem that needs thoughtful attention. It harms patients and wastes scarce healthcare resources that could be used for high-value care. It also increases spending on healthcare that could be used for education and sustainability. Many people agree that low-value care should be reduced but the crucial question is: how?

In this book, we have provided knowledge, tools, and, hopefully, inspiration to start your own project to de-implement low-value care tomorrow in your own environment. In this chapter, we will recall the lessons learned and add some practical tips for you.

*How to Reduce Overuse in Healthcare: A Practical Guide*, First Edition.
Edited by Tijn Kool, Andrea M. Patey, Simone van Dulmen, and Jeremy M. Grimshaw.
© 2024 John Wiley & Sons Ltd. Published 2024 by John Wiley & Sons Ltd.

1. *Start with choosing your own priority*
   In order to realise results on the short term, make clear what you do want to change and what you do not want to change. You cannot change the whole healthcare system. But you can start a movement in your own department, maybe in your own organisation, on a specific subject. A crucial question to begin with after you have chosen your subject is: who needs to do what differently? You should involve all relevant stakeholders for this specific subject. By involving them, they will be your ambassador during de-implementation. Reducing low-value care is easier when it is sufficiently supported by evidence and by consensus amongst healthcare professionals, for example, a professional association, or integrated in a guideline.

2. *Engage patients from the beginning*
   Patient engagement in your de-implementation intervention is more than a formal step. It can enrich your project with meaningful collaboration. A patient engagement plan is a useful tool to be explicit about how, when, and to what degree patients will be engaged. Of course, it costs time, energy, and resources, but engaging patients will increase the added value of your de-implementation intervention.

3. *Measure the low-value care and agree on a SMART target*
   Measuring the volume, rates, and variability of low-value care can help to convince your colleagues in changing their behaviour. Denial of the problem is a common defence mechanism. People will not change themselves; no one is motivated to change behaviour without external stimuli. Data can be very convincing. It gives you also the opportunity to set an improvement target. Discuss this target with all stakeholders; it should be specific, measurable, achievable, realistic, and time-bound to be accepted.

4. *Identify drivers and barriers*
   Maybe the most important phase in your de-implementation project is an analysis of which factors impede or promote the desired change. Understand why the low-value care practice you are aiming to reduce exists

and study the context of your project. This information is crucial to tailor your strategy. Take your time, without jumping to conclusions, to fully specify behaviours contributing to overuse and understand the barriers to change. It will help you to guide the selection of strategies, which may be more likely to achieve the intended impacts.

5. *Design a tailor-made strategy*
Based on the barriers and drivers you have identified, you can design your strategy. There are some frameworks, also mentioned in this book, that may help indicate which strategies are best suited to address different types of barriers. They will help you get started instead of starting from scratch. But remember, there are no magic bullets. It is important to offer acceptable alternatives.

6. *Monitor during and after the intervention*
It is very important to monitor the findings during the intervention and evaluate afterwards to determine whether your intervention has achieved the desired results. Monitoring your de-implementation intervention will ensure that it delivers what it intends to deliver, and it does not result in unintended negative consequences. Providing regular feedback about the progress can also motivate healthcare professionals in reducing overuse. A rigorous evaluation can be a good way to reassure colleagues of the importance of further reducing the low-value care practice and as a base of scaling the intervention to other departments or organisations.

7. *Start thinking right from the start how your intervention can have sustainable effects*
Even when initial de-implementation efforts are successful, interventions do not necessarily continue as originally implemented. It would be a waste if your intervention disappears unnoticed. For keeping its effects, involve staff, monitor change, use clinical leaders, and facilitate the change by, for example, a learning collaborative. You may have to seduce other colleagues to follow the movement and also change their behaviour. Your intervention will probably not sustain without specific effort.

8. *Be an ambassador for your own intervention*
It is a waste when your intervention is effective and if it is only being implemented in your own department or organisation. You might want to take a next step in scaling up. Find support for spreading your intervention, your hospital manager, your professional association, or other influential stakeholders can help you. And give other departments and organisations room for the adaption of the intervention to their local context. Their culture, beliefs, or organisational structure may be totally different from yours. You will have to respect those differences. Also, for spreading your intervention, a learning collaborative might help.

9. *Educate new healthcare professionals and those in training*
In order to reduce overuse, it is important to start changing the culture of your department. Changing existing behaviour is hard; you better start with new colleagues and residents. Give them clear instructions about the desired behaviour, for example, an open debate on the value of tests and treatments. And let the senior staff give the right example of such an open culture by stimulating a discussion between residents and staff. Educational approaches in continuous professional development activities that promote high-value care and reduce low-value practices are relevant for healthcare providers in practice as well. Examples are reflective practice and simulated communication training with a focus on behaviour and practice change.

10. *Start tomorrow*
We are sure that by reading this book, several ideas have passed your mind of how you can reduce overuse in your own environment. Do not wait and start sharing your ideas with colleagues. Realise that patients are getting harmed unnecessarily every day and scarce resources and time are being wasted. Time and money that could also be spent on high-value care. You can change that by not hesitating and starting tomorrow with a small idea that could change the culture in your organisation.

# Index

Note: *Italicized* and **bold** page numbers refer to figures and tables, respectively.

*How to Reduce Overuse in Healthcare: A Practical Guide*, First Edition.
Edited by Tijn Kool, Andrea M. Patey, Simone van Dulmen, and Jeremy M. Grimshaw.
© 2024 John Wiley & Sons Ltd. Published 2024 by John Wiley & Sons Ltd.